Gertrude's Cupboard

Recapturing Minds Stolen By Disease

E. J. Cockey

Published by E. J. Cockey and Company, P.O. Box 4132 Lutherville, Maryland 21094 www.elizabethcockey.com

Printed in the United States of America

Cover illustration by E. J. Cockey, cover design by Sherita Sparrow.

ISBN 0-9758869-1-6

Second Printing

Acknowledgments

First, I thank Nancy Gill, who encouraged me to find a new career that would benefit not only myself, but others. She took an abiding interest in my pursuit of using art as a means to recovery. And while she does not appear in this story, she was always there when I needed her the most.

Second, I thank my husband, who treated this project like his own, was there every step of the way, and became my managing editor. He made the book so much more than it was when I started..

I appreciate all the individuals who were my patients and students over the years, some of whom became my friends, and gave me advice and support for the completion of this book: Lottie Greene, Shirley Brown, Florence Herzog, Geetze Myerberg, and Elizabeth Goodhart.

I also want to thank my two sons, who stuck by me and always loved me through the good and the bad times, and who played significant roles in this story. It was through their encouragement that I decided to write and publish this book in the first place.

Lastly, but not the least, I thank Rev. Dr. Jeffrey Proctor, who taught me that good does not come to those who deserve it, but to those who are ready for it. It was through this teaching I discovered that suffering is not an inevitable part of life.

Prologue

This is a true story, about my life and the lives of those I know. Some are still with me, and some have passed away, although not everyone who passed has necessarily died. Life can be like that sometimes.

Nonetheless, I have seen fit to change the names of everyone appearing in this story, and in some cases slight identity changes have been made to protect innocent parties. I have also changed or omitted names of institutions, hospitals and long term care facilities.

I have a good friend, Linda Sue, who has a theory that people come and go. This helps her to explain the extraordinary coincidences which have led some people into her life and then right back out again. "You meet a lot of people, she told me once, but only your true friends are there to stay." And I believe what she has told me is true because even after people have come to know me well, some have stayed anyway.

I think it's always hardest in the beginning to intuit how things are going to go; as for myself, I have been fooled many times.

The author

Dedicated to

Robert S. Barber
October 7, 1922 – June 19, 2004

and

Gertrude
November 3, 1909 – July 4, 2004

Amazing grace! (how sweet the sound)
That sav'd a wretch like me!
I once was lost, but now am found,
Was blind, but now I see...

Thro' many dangers, toils and snares,
I have already come,
'Tis grace has brought me safe thus far,
And grace will lead me home.

Rev. John Newton

1779 Edition of Olney Hymns
Harry Ransom Humanities Research Center
University of Texas at Austin

"The end is always somewhere in the beginning."

Rev. Dr. Jeffrey Proctor

Chapter 1

March 2004

The phone call surprised me. It was nearly 10 pm, and I was in my studio putting the final touches on a project that was supposed to be ready for the printer on Monday morning. It was the Professor calling.

"This is Jack. I'm sorry it's late, but I wanted you to know that Gertrude has had a stroke and is in the hospital," he said. I didn't respond immediately to this bit of information because it had caught me off balance. I really didn't know what to say. Gertrude was my favorite old lady, and I felt like a part of her family. We had been together for over 5 years.

"It doesn't seem to have affected her speech; but one side of her face has gone limp, and we're not sure if she can see out of one eye," he said.

I found my voice. "Where is she now?" I asked. "She's at the hospital but will most likely be moved to another facility as soon as possible; Medicare won't let her stay once she's out of the critical care unit." All the questions that came immediately to mind seemed stupid, like was she ok, was she going to live and so forth. I knew she wasn't ok and it would probably be for the best if she did pass on; after all, what kind of life was she going to live now?

"How soon can I go see her?" I asked instead.

"Well, you can go see her anytime, once we have her placed, but she's not going to recognize you," he added. "I went to visit her today, and she thought that I was her brother Fred. Then to add insult to injury, she told me to get the hell out of her room, that this was all my fault." His voice was faltering now, and I could tell he was holding back the tears.

"The Mrs. and I have taken care of her these past six years, and at our own expense, included her in our lives and home. We've made sacrifices, and now look at all the thanks we get!" he said. His anguish was so intense I wanted to say something that would be at least somewhat comforting.

"It was very difficult when we had to place my mother in a nursing home," I said. "It's never easy, and my father felt guilty because he thought he should have been able to do something more for her."

"You know that the Mrs. promised my Dad right before he died that she would never put Gertrude in one of those places." he said. "The Mrs. is going to be devastated about this," he added. "What am I going to tell her now?"

"Look, I said, you don't have a choice anymore unless you can hire round the clock nursing care. Your wife can't possibly take care of her in this condition; we all know that." Actually, I felt that they should have placed her in a nursing center long ago. She had been going down hill for the last year. It's hard to accept that, though, when it's your own mother. I certainly understood how they felt. "We will still need you to come and do art therapy with her. It's the only nice thing she has left now," he said. "You can still go see her, can't you?"

"Don't worry, Professor; I go into those places all the time. When you know where she's going to be, just give me a call. I'll find her." I said.

"I want to thank you for all you've done for my mother over the years, and for us," he added.

"You are definitely welcome; and don't worry, I'll be there," I said. "She just wants to come home," the Professor said.

"I know, that's what everybody wants; but don't worry: I promise I'll be there for her," I said.

"Thank you again. I'll call you as soon as we know what we're going to do." We said goodbye at that point, and I hung up the phone; but I stayed up for a while after our conversation, thinking about Gertrude and what might lie ahead for her, and for her family. I remembered when my own mother had to go into a nursing facility; every time I visited she would cry and cling to me, begging me to stay, to take her home. "Please don't leave me," she would say.

Over the years I have found that while none of the histories are the same, and the afflictions vary, this is what many patients will tell me. They just want to go home. I have comforted and listened to many individuals who were living in long-term care facilities, and there are three basic questions they ask:

1) Am I going to suffer?
2) Does someone love me?
3) Did my life mean something?

Pondering these three questions and being willing to answer them has seemed to make all the difference in my life over the last several years. Ironically, the people I have worked with have helped me learn more about living than any other source ever did; for this I will always be grateful.

July 1990

Every time I stand in the cereal aisle at the grocery store I can't help but remember the summer afternoon that I stood in another aisle at the Grand Union in my home town with my mother. We were shopping together. She was looking for a particular kind of granola, and we were faced with numerous choices in a store filled with cereal. The problem was that she couldn't tell me what she wanted because she was unable to speak.

I started to point to various boxes of granola. "What do you think about the kind with raisins"? I asked. I didn't hear her say anything, so I tried again to get her attention.

"MOM!"

I got no response, and then I remembered again that she couldn't speak! I wasn't used to this scenario yet, and I was hoping she could still communicate with me. Maybe, I thought, I'll be able to read the expression on her face. I turned to look at her, but she wasn't there! Trying to suppress panic, I looked down the aisle to see if mother was anywhere in sight. She was standing by the dairy case, picking up yogurt and cottage cheese from the display. She had several containers of each and was carefully placing them into someone else's cart. Our own cart was still a little bit behind me on my left.

"Good Lord!" I said. She looked up from the stranger's cart, saw me, then pointed in my direction and started giggling. I turned around in time to see what she was pointing at. It was her closest neighbor, Jean Brown, who was approaching us. My mother's affliction was not something my family wanted everybody in town to find out about. This was a secret that we had decided to keep, and right now it was up to me to maintain security. What was worse, Mrs. Brown was the biggest busybody in town. I thought she had really missed her calling by not writing a gossip column for the local newspaper.

I put on my happiest face and was smiling at her as she maneuvered her cart my way. But she ignored me completely and walked down the aisle towards my Mother. "How are you, Annette?" she said to my mother. "I heard you were in the hospital!"

Mother was still somewhat giggly, but to my great relief, she didn't respond. Instead of saying anything she pushed the cart she had been putting yogurt into around the corner, disappearing behind a canned goods display. I couldn't believe it! How was I ever going to keep this secret, and how did Mrs. Brown find out so soon about my mother? Before I could think about a reasonable excuse for her behavior, Mrs. Brown had moved closer to me and in a hushed voice asked me for details. Her eyes were wide with surprise and delight.

"What was the diagnosis?" she whispered.

"Gee, I don't know; the jury's still out," I lied. My brain was working fast now. "But poor Mom caught something while she was in the hospital, and now she's got laryngitis. She's not supposed to be using her voice today. Also I think she's a bit confused with all the commotion."

"That's terrible!" Mrs. Brown's face was all scrunched up, and I could tell that she was sizing up my story, wondering what to do with this information. I kept quiet, wondering whether she would begin to interrogate me if I hung around any longer. But she didn't say anything, and I felt more confident that I had managed to stay on top of the situation.

"Well, stay in touch," she said, "and don't be a stranger."

"I'm only here for a few more days," I said. To indicate that our conversation had reached a conclusion, I pushed my cart around Mrs. Brown, making a bee line for the canned goods, where I was relieved to find my mother. She was examining cans of peas, Delmonte Peas, Green Giant Peas, and so forth.

"Let's get out of here", I said. "Please Mom, before anyone else sees us!" I think I must have surprised her because the next thing that she did really got me. To this very day it still bothers me. Mother started to cry, loudly enough that everyone within a short distance could hear her. Tears were running down her face.

"Let's go home," I said frantically. "Let's just forget the stupid cereal." She stopped crying for a moment as if she were pondering this, then reached out to clutch my hand with hers. She has never liked it when I get upset. And so, fortunately we were able to make our way out the door like that, abandoning the cart, with me holding on to her arm, and her clutching mine. I managed to propel her like that towards the lot where I had parked the car. It was difficult and awkward. The sun was bearing down, and it was hot.

I thought that I should say something that might calm her and that indirectly would calm me too, which is how I came to say to her that it was going to be all right somehow. "It's going to be ok, this is nothing! Why I've seen worse than this!" I said. She didn't respond, except to begin shaking and crying again. I didn't know what to do. Interestingly I remember that my main thought was about myself, not her. How could I take mother anywhere anymore, not knowing what she might do next? Her actions might embarrass me! What would our friends think? It seemed that the only thing I could do now was to take her home. That was my answer that afternoon. She was going home, and I was taking her there. Mother was going to live there with my father, and she was going to get better! It was going to be ok. It was. I was going to insist on it!

My parents had retired earlier that same year, and had decided to build their dream house down by the river on some property that had been part of the family farm. Actually, the land hadn't been farmed for at least a generation; so the riverfront property was an ideal location for a peaceful way of life. Their new home was a rustic cabin, with a cedar deck around it, and you could hear a chorus of animal sounds from every direction. They were going to be happy there; they had planned it that way. But it never worked out the way they had planned.

Several days before the actual completion of the house, my mother had suffered a grand mal seizure while she was swimming laps at the YWCA. She was always an active person and had planned to stay that way by exercising on a daily basis. Mother's favorite activity was swimming, and she did twenty laps every day. On this particular day, though, she had dived into the pool and hadn't come up, not until she was noticed on the bottom and was dragged up to the side by one of the lifeguards. An ambulance was called, and she was taken to the hospital immediately. Later, a CAT scan revealed that there were angiomas in her brain, little knots of abnormal blood vessels that had caused the seizure and consequently her loss of speech and slight dementia. Despite all this, the Doctor was reassuring." Don't worry; in a few days she'll be right as rain," he said.

So, my mother was sent home with a bottle full of anti-seizure medication and was told to relax. Yet, it wasn't until another year had gone by, and after many other tests and trips to the hospital that the final diagnosis was made. Mother had been born with a very rare hereditary disorder, familial cerebral angiomatosis. The lesions in her brain had grown larger as she had grown older, until the day that one of them ruptured in the left frontal lobe, robbing her of speech. Eventually these same lesions also robbed her of a relationship with my father, their dream house on the river, and the ability to take care of herself.

To his credit, my father took care of her all by himself in the new house for the next five years. When questioned about this decision he replied, "I promised I wouldn't send her to a nursing home." But one day while he was out shopping, mother fell in the bathroom and lay in her urine, confused and frightened, for several hours until my father came home. She had gotten herself wedged between the toilet and the wall. Their dog Yankee was licking her face. My father found her, and she didn't remember who he was.

She doesn't remember me now either, or any of us for that matter: my sister and brother, our children, or her friends. She was moved to the Alzheimer's unit last Spring. I've been advised by the Doctor not to call anymore on the phone because it upsets her, and she cries. She thinks I am coming to take her home again.

But home is just not the same without her being there; so I don't visit more than twice a year. I don't like to admit it, but I just can't stand it. When I do visit I have to see her in the special care unit at Community Convalescent Home. It is devastating to see her in a wheelchair, to be unable to talk with her, and to have to leave her behind when I go. The last time I saw my Mother, all she said was this: "Don't leave me!"

"So, when Jane asked me how I did it, I told her, I just paint what I see!"

Gertrude

Chapter 2

The hospital has a nursing facility behind the main building, and it is one of my favorite places to practice art as a therapy. The activity room is on the second floor and has tall windows on three sides which look out onto a tree lined street below. There is ample light and lots of space to move wheel chairs around without bumping into someone. Appropriately, it's called the Park Unit. If you are deaf, Park Unit is a good place to hang out during the day. Otherwise with all the noises, both mechanical and human, you could really consider being deaf an asset. There are bells ringing and beepers beeping and little old ladies and men strapped into wheelchairs and half beds, who stare up at the ceiling and repeat the same things over and over and over all day long, every day, perpetually.

"Mommy, mommy, mommy, mommy." . . . ." one lady cries.

March 2003

I step off the elevator and turn right at the doors. Alex has already set up the room by moving tables together and covering them with plastic cloths. A group of nurses' aides help Alex move the patients around the room and into place at the tables as I arrive. For at least another 5 minutes there is a bustle of activity, and once everyone is rounded up there are 16 people ready to begin Art class. I work with, more or less, the same group of individuals every week. Sometimes a person dies, but that's about the only reason they don't show up on a regular basis to paint with me.

They are bored.

Truth be told there's not a lot of activities you can do with a mixed bag of people, suffering from a wide variety of neurological diseases such as Parkinson's, Alzheimer's disease, dementia, and MS. There are also other Special needs residents here in the nursing facility: amputees, diabetics, and quadriplegics.

The reason I came to Park Unit in the first place was to see if I could help this same group of residents because they were clinically depressed. The reason they were depressed was that they were spending the rest of their lives on Park Unit, minus arms and legs and minds. They were all having normal reactions to their monotonous and institutionalized living conditions.

"Let's do art!" I announce, as I walk to the end of one of the tables and wait for their attention.

E. J. Cockey

I stand next to Betty, who lost a leg last year to diabetes and has been in a wheelchair ever since. She is wearing a bright green plastic party hat which is left over from a St. Patrick's Day celebration the night before. One hand is strapped down to her wheelchair in some kind of foam contraption. In the other hand she holds a short stick with a coat hook attached to one end by duct tape. Betty eyeballs me from her ground position and gets a look on her face that tells me something's coming.

"Git her outta here!" she bellows and points to Mary, who is sitting a couple of seats down from her.

"Hey", I say, "what's up with the big stick, Betty? Aren't they feeding you this week?" This comment brings laughter from Betty's end of the table. Then I turn to the object of Betty's wrath, a lady of undeterminable age, also in a wheelchair. I tend to agree with Betty that this lady is, in her terms, "a total pain in the ass."

"Hey Mary", "I say, "How are you today?"

"I can't find my glasses, and my head hurts so much that I can't paint," Mary whines.

"Knock it off, Mary", I say. "You never can find your glasses. Why heck, I don't think you even own glasses!" Several of the other patients laugh at this too, and one lady named Helen tells me that Mary is definitely lying.

"Yes I do, but SHE probably took them," Mary says, sneering and pointing at Betty.

"She was born with a headache!"

"Was not!"

Sitting next to Mary is a gentleman named Darren. He is 79 years old and suffers from advanced dementia. I first met Darren 4 years ago. He was sitting in the same seat that he occupies now; only now he is looking around the room and smiling, waiting patiently to become the next person I "pick on". He likes to reminisce about the time he started painting with me. We go over this story every week or so. I clap him on the shoulder.

"Hey buddy, what's up!"

"Stop messin'ith me," Darren says.

"I'm here especially to mess with you!" I remind him.

"Remember when I threw that brush?"

"Darren, you threw that brush 3 or 4 times across this room, and I picked it up every time and handed it back to you!"

"And then I painted the pumpkin," he says.

"And you haven't stopped painting yet!" I add. He smiles and looks down at his hands.

Actually, Darren sat at the activity table for a couple of years, refusing to do anything. He didn't interact with others, and he didn't like to be disturbed. He preferred to sit and face the tall windows on Park Unit. Trouble was that he didn't even look out at the scenery, but sat with his face pointing down all day and everyday. Apparently the art class was the first social program that had any effect upon him at all.

Betty has an electric wheelchair which she has just maneuvered into place at the head of the table. She is the alpha-female at Park Unit. She is also my favorite. I just love her stick with the coat hanger on the end. She invented the contraption to push the button on the elevator since her hands don't reach from the wheelchair. She's a survivor.

"Come here!" she calls to me.

"What now?" I reply.

"I gotta tell you sompin' what I said." She has that same gleam in her eye, and I wonder what story she has for me this time.

Usually her language and her manner are rather crude, but she has a wonderful sense of humor. I look around the unit as I make my way over to her, checking to see if any family members are hanging around or anyone else who might be offended by what I anticipate will be a graphic description. She grabs a hold of my arm and pulls me down until my head is on the same level as hers.

"Wanna know what I told the aide at lunch today?" she asks. She sits back now and waits for me to respond. There is a naughty look on her face now.

"No, what?"

"So, I told her, you git over here and take this lousy sandwich back to the kitchen. You smelled this thing, I said to her? And she says she ain't smelt nothing today 'cause she's so busy. So I says to her, well you just git your nose down here cause I'm telling you this thing smells worse than my pussy does!" She sits back in her chair laughing and waiting for my reaction.

I whisper into her ear, cupping my hand around the side of her head so no one else will hear. "You really need to find yourself a dancing partner."

"Trouble is, there ain't no booty around anywhere worth having." she says. Betty laughs again loudly and then raps her stick on the table. This is the signal that the class should come to order, because she does this every week. It's a ritual. All sixteen sets of eyes are on me.

"Let's paint, folks."

The next phase is all about movement and confusion mixed in with a little patience, some fighting and a lot of laughter. Let me explain. There are always 15 to 20 individuals present for the Art class, and they have been clustered around the tables with some space in between, so that I can squeeze in between them.

Generally they have a tendency not to socialize with one another unless they are playing bingo.

There are other people assisting me today: Alex, the activity aide; Chris, my personal assistant; Sister Maria, a Sister of Charity; and usually a random family member. Today there are two men flanking a lady named Ernestine: William and Stan. I can tell by their faces that they desperately want Ernestine to participate in this activity. She's new to the Park Unit, and it's very normal for people's families to want to get them off to a great start. It eases the pain they feel when they have to go home and leave their Grandma or their spouse behind.

"Why don't you stay where you are and paint with her?" I tell them.

"You sure it wouldn't be no trouble?" William asks. "I'm her husband."

"Of course not, I'll have Alex bring you some paper."

Alex is already handing out white paper to everyone and Chris is distributing paint brushes. I head for the paint cart and begin to squirt different colors into small plastic drinking cups. Betty is working on an outdoor scene with azaleas in bloom. One of the assistants has given her the wrong color, and she has painted a stream in with gray instead of light blue.

"This looks like shit" she complains.

"Hold tight Betty; I'll be right with you." I reply.
I decide to give Sue the blue paint first. She is sitting on Betty's right and has a big sky area that could be filled in nicely with this particular hue. I figure that Betty can use it in a minute. They will have to learn how to share. Instead Sue looks up at me and whines "I hate that color."

"Knock it off, Sue; this is an awesome color for that sky." She grudgingly takes the cup and starts to fill in the top of her painting, a landscape. "I want to paint a horse instead," she says.

"OK, but not now!" I tell her.

Mary is next. Her arms are crossed, and she announces that she's only watching today. "I've got a bad headache today!" she says.

"That's wonderful, darling!"

"My stomach hurts too!" I know that she is only saying this because she needs the attention. I give her one of my stern looks while Alex hands her a cup of red paint. I must add that I am not trying to be mean to anyone. But this is therapy, and they are here to begin using arms and hands again. Talking and laughter come next, sometimes in a few weeks, usually in several months, but they always come.

For this I give thanks.

This activity lasts 1 ½ hours. I had to increase the time from the typical hour I usually allow for disabled individuals. So many people wanted to come and paint that we scarcely had time to give everyone the attention they deserved. It would seem as if we had just gotten started when it would be quitting time. So, we added some time and now we're off to the races! In fact the activity director has told me that my art class is as popular as bingo!

Finally they settle down, and everyone is painting, with the exception of Rosie, who is sleeping. She's still holding onto a brush full of brown paint even though she is slumped over in her wheelchair. I sigh. I'm tired and everyone seems moody today.   I look up to see what time it is; already 45 minutes have gone by.

Where does the time go?

I look out the windows for a moment, watching the clouds drift by, hearing the traffic sounds on Smith Avenue: cars braking, horns blowing and people calling to each other down below. The yelling reminds me of another time, and I let my mind drift as I stare out the window.

August 1956

The main thing I remember about my grandmother is that she was the ruler of our family, the sustainer and law-giver; and the family's feeling of security depended upon her. She was a devout Baptist and completely opposed to the enjoyment of life's pleasures, abstaining from many things: the consumption of alcohol, playing cards, wearing makeup, touching, dancing, singing, laughing. She felt that it was her job to see to it that none of us strayed too far from the arms of *Jesus!* Poor Grandmother had had to grow up when she was about 9 years old. Her own mother, Sarah, was sickly and took to her bed about 1904. So, the running of the house, cooking for the men, cleaning, and looking after her little brother filled up Fanny's days, nights, and the remainder of her childhood years and formed the pattern of her adult life.

Anyway, one gray and moody August afternoon when I was 5 years old, I had climbed up on top of the kitchen counter where I could sit in the large, enameled sink. It was directly in front of the kitchen window, giving me a great view of the barn. I was looking at the barn from the sink, my face pressed to the glass, thinking about horses. My grandfather had promised to buy me a horse when I was old enough, and I daydreamed about riding them all the time.

There was a dense stillness in the air outside; the birds had stopped chirping, the wind had stopped, and the sky had turned gray. The wind picked up and blew puffs of dust across the driveway in front of our house.

Suddenly my daydreaming was interrupted by a huge BOOM, as a large hand of fire reached right down into the top of our barn followed by an immense CRACK and then another BOOM ! Almost immediately flames roared up and out of the roof. Lightning had struck the haymow, and the barn was burning!

The next thing I saw was my Grandfather running across the lawn. He had his tall black rubber boots on. I called them his shit kicker boots because he always wore them to muck out the stalls.

I remember wondering why he had those boots on. I just didn't see what difference they would make to a fire.

He was screaming to my father, who followed close behind him. "Get moving; the barn is on fire!"

My father hurried faster, toward the flames. He was carrying a three pronged hay fork. I thought he looked like a picture of Lucifer, the devil that I had seen in Sunday school. My father the devil, a disturbing thought. I had been instructed that Lucifer was the ultimate bad guy.

Meanwhile, a different kind of calamity had taken over our household. My stalwart Baptist grandmother had come completely undone. She was running all over the place crying and carrying on and upsetting everyone. My mother was screaming too; my baby brother was crying; and my little sister was whining that she was hungry. I, on the other hand, had remained at my perch on the kitchen sink where I had an extremely good view of the fire and the goings-on. I was yet unnoticed and hadn't been missed by the adults with all the excitement of the fire.

Phone calls must have been made, because it wasn't too long before the townspeople started to arrive and parked on the lawn, either to help or to watch the 150-year- old barn burn to the ground. Pretty soon the driveway and the front lawn had filled up with their cars. Some of the farm women had come along with their husbands and had found my Grandmother sobbing on the steps, just under my window perch.

"We're ruined!" she cried.

I remember about 5 or 6 women hovering around her, like a football huddle. All heads were pointed towards the ground, and I supposed that they were praying for the barn to stop burning. Eventually our minister, the Reverend Charles Plummer, appeared in the midst of this group of ladies. He was carrying two juice glasses, filled to the middle with a light brown liquid. He pulled up a lawn chair and sat directly in front of my grandmother, who was starting to cry again and rocking back and forth.

"Fanny Barber", he said, "you are going to pull yourself together now, and we are going to pray." She kept right on sobbing. He tried again.

"Here, sit up and drink this down." he commanded her. She looked up and took the juice glass in her hand.

"Just wha.. what am I d..drink..drinking?" she sobbed.

"It's medicine for the soul."

She sniffed the contents of the glass and sat up straight. Her voice was suddenly commanding again "Oh law, it's alcohol, the work of the devil!" she cried.

The next thing he told her has stuck with me ever since. "Sometimes we just have to make exceptions." he said. Then, the Reverend drained his glass in one long gulp. He set the glass down on the ground and waited.

"Am I going to go to Hell for drinking this?" Her hand was shaking, and some of the liquid was spilling out. He steadied her hand. "If you're going to Hell, then I'm going right there with you!" he said. So she took a breath, and she drank the stuff all the way down.

"You are CRAZY!" was all she said afterwards.

March, 2003

A sudden splash interrupts my thoughts, and I am brought back to reality. A tiny lady named Clarabelle has accidentally knocked a glass of juice onto the floor. She is 97 years old and is so small that she can barely reach the top of the table. One of the nurses' aides comes to the rescue with a towel to mop up.

I hurry over and stand next to Clarabelle. She is crying. I lean over and put my arms around her. She is all bones, everywhere; so she's hard to hug. I squeeze her anyway "I'm so sorry", she says.

"SO WHAT!" I tell her. "It doesn't matter; we can get you some more juice!"

But let me explain myself before I go any further. This story will make more sense if I supply some sort of context to hang it all on. Writing is a lot like the art I do with dementia patients. I give them a context by drawing a line to form a particular shape: it could be a house, a tree, a vase or the street below. It's always clear what I'm talking about that way. A tree is a tree, after all

I started working about 8 years ago as an art teacher for several long term care facilities. At first I worked with dementia and Alzheimer's patients, later expanding to include others with special needs and others who were depressed. I'm one of the people who care for individuals our society has cast aside: the ones who need us the most; the dying, the infirm, and the meek.

The story I'm telling lies in the experience we have had together. Me, on the outside looking in. Them on the inside, pushing out. In retrospect, I think that I have brought laughter to them, but what they have given me is much greater. I found out that we are not equal, none of us. Some ride in wheelchairs; others can't see. Many are crippled and incontinent with leaky brains, dead limbs, useless bodies. They are multicolored. Some are still young, most are very old. Many are forgotten. The truth is we are all uniquely different, not the same. But what they have taught me is that we are something far more important than equal.

We are all in this together. Let me back up then and tell this story when it really begins, starting when I met Gertrude.

Chapter 3

The first time I met Gertrude, she was only 88 years old. She lived with her son and his family in the nicest part of town. The street was lined with elms that had withstood the blight of the 50's and 60's. Dappled light shone down through their leaves in the warm months and cast elegant shadows in the winter. In the tidy neighborhood pond were ducks with duck babies, and around it strolled women with human babies.

Gertrude's family lived in a looming stone house, built in 1926 at the top of a hill, with a hundred steps leading up to the front door. At first it reminded me of a castle because it was covered with vines. The house had old azaleas and well established perennials growing along its borders. Whenever I walk up the steps I always remember the wonderful dampness and green smells that greeted me that first day, before I went inside for an interview.
I spoke with the Professor and his wife in their living room, mostly about my credentials, work experience, and fee schedule.

They told me that their mother had been living with them since her husband had died, and she had become severely depressed. The visiting nurse who worked for them had advised they seek an art or music therapist to work with Gertrude since the antidepressants had failed to lift her spirits.

"Do you think you can help my mother?" the Professor asked.

"I'll certainly give it my best, sir." I said.

"Fine, fine", he said, "Shall we go upstairs and meet her then?"

"Oh yes, sir, I would love to do that."

Gertrude lived on the second floor. Her bedroom was over the garage; so it was hot in the summer and cold in the winter. Her only window looked out into the alley behind the house. Her transient companions in the alley were the neighborhood cats, dogs and squirrels on a regular basis and the city garbage collectors on Mondays and Thursdays.

Breakfast, lunch and dinner are delivered to Gertrude's room on a tray. She has had the same breakfast *and* lunch every day, for the last 3 years. I don't know about dinner. Of course it is not like that all the time. On special holidays and birthdays her family lugs her down stairs, and she eats with them in the dining room, just like normal.

Every once in a while I would convene with Gertrude's family about her well-being and whatever progress we had made. The meetings were difficult to schedule with them. The Mrs. volunteered at the Museum (a lot) and the Professor was a research scientist who frequently traveled around the world. They were always very busy, but they were also trying to do what they thought was right for their Mother. God Bless them for trying.

A maid cleaned the house; a visiting nurse specialist checked her vital signs, and an aide came every other day to bathe and dress her. I came on Mondays and Thursdays for an hour to do the activities. But she was still depressed, and they couldn't understand WHY! So we continued to have these meetings. I told them that Gertrude needed more stimulation, and they told me that I made a difference in her life.

"You have absolutely extended my Mother's life," the Professor told me one time. "Thank you from the bottom of my heart!"

November 1999

Gertrude has told me her whole life story in bits and pieces over the years. Fortunately she repeats herself all the time; so I have inadvertently memorized every detail. The first time I met Gertrude, her son the Professor took me upstairs and then down a long dark hallway to her room. He knocked gently at the door before entering. The room was as dark as the hall that led up to it. It was a small room filled to the brim with big furniture. There was a couch on one side piled with stacks of laundry, and two chests on different walls; one had a mirror hanging at the top and the other one had a big television set on it. The television was on, but Gertrude wasn't watching. She was sitting at a wiggly card table and sorting photographs into piles.

Her son spoke tentatively. "Mother, I have someone here to see you!" When she didn't look up, he tried again, louder. "Mother, someone is here to visit with you today!"

"What did you say?" She said.

"I have the art teacher with me, and she wants to meet you." he said.

"I don't paint anymore, can't see right; get out of here." she said.

He tried again. "Mother, the art teacher is right here and she"........but Gertrude cut him off in mid-sentence.
"I'm NOT painting; I'm old!" she replied. Right about then his pager started beeping. He turned towards me, and he said, "I'll step out and let you two get to know each other now.

I'll be down in my study if you need me." Then he was out the door, and I stood facing her, alone.

"Hi, I guess you already know that I'm an artist," I said. "May I sit down?"

"Suit yourself, but I'm not painting today. I'm sorting through my things."

"Why don't you let me help?" I asked. I glanced around and found a straight-backed chair that I pulled over to the card table where she was sitting.

"This is about all I've got left of my memories," she said without looking up. "They don't let me have any of my own furniture since I'm in such cramped quarters. After my husband died, they came and got me, and I've been in this room ever since."

"How long have you been here, Gertrude?" I asked.

"I just told you, since my husband died." And with that she sat back and jutted her jaw out at me.

"I was thinking in terms of days and months," I said.

"Eight months, more or less," she replied. "And why do you care to know anyway? You don't even know me."

Initial meetings have always been difficult for me. What does one say to a person who is having a healthy response to tough circumstances? "Hello, I'm going to make this all better for you?" Instead, I leaned closer to her. "Your family thought you might like to start some art lessons," I said. "I'm your entertainment, so to speak."

"I used to paint with the nuns," she said. "It was a long time ago." Then she pushed her wheelchair back a bit and reached over to an old dresser that had many drawers. She started pulling out the drawers and examining the contents in several of them. Finally, after rummaging through the drawers, she found what she was looking for.

"Ah ha! This is the first painting I ever did! The nun used to say to me, "just paint what you see, Gertrude; just paint what you see!" She sat back in her chair and smiled broadly. In her lap she held a small canvas board that had an autumn landscape painted on it, evidence that she had in fact painted before.

"That's wonderful," I said. But I was more interested in the dresser behind her that was full of drawers, the contents of which held a great interest for me. When she started opening the drawers, I had glimpsed that in some there were bright materials or maybe buttons, letters and underwear all mixed up together and all packed into little compartments, representing the different directions her life had taken. "My goodness", I said to her, "it's your mother's dresser."

"No it's not, it's my cupboard," she replied.

"It looks like an old dresser to me," I said.

Gertrude scowled at me from her wheelchair. "Now just what is it that you are doing here?" she asked.

"I'll be coming back on Monday to teach you how to paint," I said. She frowned again. "I just got through showing you; I already know how to paint!" she said.

"Yes, thank you Gertrude; and I'll be seeing you Monday," I said. Then I was out the door, back down the dark hall and the two flights of stairs. If the Professor was still in his study, he was being very quiet. I didn't feel like taking up any more of my time, so I slipped silently out the back door, got in my car and began the long drive home. Gertrude's family and I had already agreed upon a contractual arrangement for the next six months. It was good money. I needed the money, and Gertrude needed me. Driving past the ponds and the big houses, I asked myself *what does someone say to a person who is suffering?*

There is only one thing you can say, and it is this: "You are going to get better!"

'Twas grace that taught my heart to fear, and grace my fears reliev'd

Rev. John Newton

Chapter 4

November 1999

Fall had finally arrived, and the weather had been crisp during the day; but this particular evening it had begun to drizzle, and it seemed darker than usual for the ride home. I was later than normal getting into traffic because of the interview with Gertrude; so by the time I got on the beltway there was a bottleneck of cars and big trucks all trying to squeeze into two lanes going north.

I had just moved to an old, rambling farmhouse about 30 minutes out of town. It was in the county, a place that was more of a hamlet than a town. The house stood at the intersection of two roads. It was nearly 200 years old and in the old days had served as an inn for travelers on the way to Baltimore. At some point in the house's life someone had remodeled, and nothing they had done was historically accurate. There was an old livery stable that still stood in great disrepair on the front end of the property, but that was the only building that remained as it had been from the earlier part of the century. My landlady had bought the place at a foreclosure auction. She said that in a couple of years she hoped to save up enough money to have the stable torn down before it fell down. The house was a bit run down, and the yard was overgrown; but it was my idea of semi-retirement to the country, where I could relax and do some landscape painting in relative peace and quiet.

The drive was longer than if I had remained in the suburbs, but I was getting used to it. I had turned on the radio to listen to the news and the weather report. It was nearly Thanksgiving, and outside my car window the drizzle was transforming into slushy rain/snow. It was becoming harder for me to see the road, and I was approaching another part of the highway where several more lanes of traffic would be merging.

The traffic was barely moving now, and cars were creeping forward at about ten miles an hour. My lane had completely stopped; so I was playing with the radio dials and waiting. All of a sudden, I felt the rear end of my car rise, as if lifted by some unseen and alien force.

"What is going on!" I yelled. I turned to look out my window and gasped. I was looking directly into the lettering on a door of a Mack truck; all the while the back end of my car was being lifted off the ground.

"What is happening?" I cried in desperation.

The truck had gotten too close to my little sports car, and the lug nuts of the truck's wheels had gotten stuck under the fender of my car. When the truck went forward, the left side of my car was jacked up off the ground. Worse yet, the driver of the truck hadn't even seen me and my little car because of the wet darkness. I needed to take quick action or be crushed under the wheels of the tractor trailer.

I shifted into first gear and stepped on the gas, hoping to break away. I gave it more gas, and the car wiggled from side to side for a moment. My heart was in my throat. I shifted again into second gear and once more slammed my foot on the gas. I heard a loud ripping sound, smelled burned rubber and then felt the car drop down to the ground again before bumping forward. Traffic had started to move again too; and the trucker, oblivious to me, was rolling away down the road. I could just barely make out something hanging from the side of his truck. I didn't dare look around or stop to evaluate the damage to my car because the traffic was moving faster now, and I was afraid I'd be killed on the side of the road if I stopped. I drove all the way home like that, with a sense of apprehension. I just couldn't shake it. It felt like an ominous prediction of things to come.

When I pulled up into the driveway, the back porch lights came on, and my landlady rushed out the door to greet me. "Oh my God!" was what she said, but the look on her face told me everything.

I slowly climbed out of the car and turned around for my own look. The entire back panel had been ripped off the car, and the bumper was hanging down to the ground on the driver's side. "I'm just a wreck!" was what I said to her. I was trying to be funny, but I just couldn't pull it off.

"Oh my God!" she said again. "Let me give you a big hug!"

I held my hand up, keeping her at arms length. "I don't want a big hug; I need a drink!"

So we went inside where it was warm. She had made a fire in the fireplace, and I followed in behind her. "I heated up some of the vegetable soup," she said. "Would you like some?"

"Do I have to get it myself?" I asked. She didn't say anything, so I had a moment to think about what I did want. "Never mind, I said to her, I'm gonna make that drink instead." I went downstairs to where the kitchen was located. The old house was built into a hill, and since it had once served as an inn, the kitchen and the washroom were "downstairs" along with a couple of bedrooms for the domestic help. She lived downstairs, and I lived upstairs. She had a kitchen, and I had a room with a view.

Tonight, though, I felt as if I were trespassing into her domain. I felt weird in there, looking through her cabinets for a bottle of bourbon. I finally found it. It was hidden behind a pile of plastic Tupperware containers that had fallen down inside the cupboard.

It was like looking through the contents of someone's personal things after they have died. I knew that the Tupperware had come from a time when she had been married. She hadn't worked then; she'd stayed home and made babies, hung drapes, and cooked delicious dinners for her husband. Now all the stuff she had accumulated during her marriage was either packed in boxes in the attic or stuffed into the cupboards in the kitchen. She had supplemented her income by renting out rooms to transient people, roommates all, never relationships that lasted for very long.

It was sad to be standing in the kitchen, holding on to a bottle of liquor and knowing there was a warm fire upstairs and the comfort of a roommate waiting for me. But I didn't feel like going upstairs. I remained alone, drinking straight from the bottle. Standing there in her kitchen was like standing in the middle of someone else's life, where every moment had been put away forever, out of sight, in the cupboards. I had cleaned out my own apartment before moving into this house with her. I had hired an estate sales person, who packed up almost everything I owned and auctioned it all off. She had given me a check for 2000 dollars, and I had moved into Evelyn's house with my clothes, art supplies, my computer, and some paintings.

I was depressed all of a sudden. When I really thought about it, I was much worse off than even old Gertrude. She at least had hung onto her memories, by placing everything meaningful in her cupboard; but I had thrown mine away. Now my car was trashed too. I wasn't even certain I could drive to work or anywhere for that matter. Finally, with that realization, I sat down on the cold stone floor in Evelyn's kitchen and cried.

I woke up the next morning with the sound of rain against my window. I could hear some birds chirping and the din of music being played somewhere on a lower floor of the house. I had taken a few too many drinks the night before but had somehow managed to climb the three flights of stairs to my room, dropped onto the top of my bed, and passed out. I hadn't gotten under the covers either; so I was still dressed in the same clothes that I had worn to work the day before. My head was throbbing, and I was thirsty.

It was like coming out of a bad dream, and I was trying to remember what time it was and what had happened. Then I remembered about my car. *"Oh no!"* It was the day before Thanksgiving, and I knew that it might be difficult to get in touch with my insurance agent, much less get a rental car.

I looked around for my watch to see what time it was. My alarm clock had been mistakenly sold off by the estate liquidator, and I hadn't replaced it yet. I figured it must be going on noon. With this thought I bolted straight out of bed and ran down the hall. I yelled, "What time is it?

Evelyn hollered back, "Eleven thirty!"

"I might need to borrow your car!" I yelled, then moved to the top of the stairs so I wouldn't have to continue to yell. My head hurt.

"When do you need it?" she asked, "I've got to pick up Micky at noon from his school." She was standing at the bottom of the stairs that led up to the third floor in an old pink terry cloth robe, holding a cup of coffee in one hand and a cigarette in the other. Micky was her 11 year old son, and he attended a private Christian school somewhere in the county. His real name was Michael Bennett Skinner, III, but Evelyn hadn't gotten out of the habit of calling him the nickname Micky since he was a baby. I felt sorry for him.

"If I leave now I can be back here by 1:30," she said.

"I need to pick up Gray at the airport by three;" I said. "Will I have enough time to get to the airport from here?"

"Oh God, yes!" she replied.

"You're not going to drive to that school dressed like that are you?" I asked.

"Like WHAT?"

"In that bathrobe," I said. I felt it should have been more obvious to her.

"Looked into the mirror lately?" she asked. And with that remark she tapped the long ash of her cigarette into the pot of a very dried-up plant that occupied a corner near the stairs. Sometimes she could be really disgusting. I even thought she did it to me on purpose once in a while. Anyway, she disappeared into her room, and I could hear her moving things around. About 2 minutes later, she was bounding down the stairs. I heard the slam of the back door and her car starting up and then the crunch of gravel.

I walked back down the hallway to my bathroom and looked into the mirror. It was an old mirror that was probably installed sometime in the 1930's. There were places around the edges where the back of the mirror had gone dark, and so it didn't reflect anything there. Consequently, parts of my hairline were missing at the top of the mirror. There was a flaw that ran from top to bottom, causing a wavelike imperfection down the middle. My reflection looked like a picture taken with a wide angle lens. I looked terrible. The dark circles under my eyes were darker than usual, and my hair was bushy.

I looked out the bathroom window to the driveway behind the house. There was my little sports car, with one side hanging, nearly ripped off the frame. In comparison, I was still of the opinion that I looked worse than the car. I was going to have to take a shower, and that was all there was to it. After all, the show must go on; my son was expecting me to pick him up at the airport later that afternoon.

After about 30 minutes, I'd showered and dressed and was drinking a cup of coffee, waiting for Evelyn to return and the insurance people to call me back. The insurance company called first. The insurance lady had it all figured out; I was supposed to drop my sports car off at the body shop for an estimate, and the rental car people would meet me. But best of all, I got to arrange the details of all this around my trip to the airport. The other good news was that I didn't have to wait around for Evelyn to show up because now I didn't have to borrow her car. Suddenly I felt relieved. I wasn't at the effect of anything now! Not one. But that feeling didn't last long. Just about then my phone rang again. I answered it after the second ring.

"Hallo," I said.

"It's John," he said. I was taken slightly by surprise at hearing his deep baritone voice again. We hadn't talked in nearly six months, not since our son had gotten married. Suddenly I was troubled. John is my sons' father, and I was worried that our youngest kid had missed his plane. He lived with John in San Antonio, and he was supposed to be on a Southwest Airlines flight right now, eating peanuts.

"Gray's flight isn't delayed, is it?" I asked. There was a pause and then his voice was not so melodious or resounding.

"No, that's not why I called. Ben's tried to kill himself."

I was certain I hadn't heard him correctly. "What did you say, John? I couldn't hear you very well; radio's turned on." I reached over and turned the radio off so that I could hear what he was saying.

"I SAID that Ben tried to take his LIFE yesterday afternoon," he said.

I sat down on the floor. It felt as if the air had gone out of me, but on the other hand I couldn't feel any emotion about what he had just told me concerning our oldest son, either. It was a rather strange sensation. I can only liken the experience to an anxiety attack when there is a terrible lack of air, a feeling of suffocation. There I was on the floor of my room, looking under my bed, where the dust balls hadn't had time to form yet. It was sad and it was strange to know all these things, on the eve of Thanksgiving, I involuntarily shuddered and remembered the last time we all were together. I looked at my watch to see what time it was. It was nearly 1 pm, and I had to leave for the airport. Now I felt another urgency somehow handling the plethora of things to do before driving home again in a different car, possibly in the dark.

My son had tried to take his life! I remembered when he was happy.

June 1999

Ben had met Debby in the fall of 1998, at a restaurant where they both worked. He was a chef, and she managed the front. They had dated briefly. One day he hadn't shown up for work, and after a while Debby had gone to look for him. After quite a long hunt, she found Ben underneath his bed, in his apartment where he seemed to be unconscious but in fact was having a grand mal seizure. He had been missing for 24 hours, but no one knew how long he had been under the bed. So they rushed him to the hospital.

There were a lot of exams while he was there, but nothing was conclusive. Five little bleeds in his brain had showed up on a CAT scan, though, and it was suggested he go in for more extensive testing at Johns Hopkins Hospital's neurology department. We were standing in his room at the hospital, deciding how to transport Ben over to Hopkins when Debby came in. She looked somewhat nervous and said that she had something important to tell us. We stopped talking for a moment to listen to what she had to say.

"I'm pregnant," she announced.

He never made it to Hopkins. Instead they decided to get engaged and drive to Florida because she wanted to be near her family when she had the baby. In spite of my protests, Ben sold his car to buy her a diamond ring, and they drove off in her Toyota near the end of February.

I flew to Naples, Florida with my best friend Elliot in mid-June for the wedding. The service took place in a fancy hotel down by the sea, and the bride's family had decorated extravagantly. The wedding pictures were taken at dusk. The sky was peach and lavender, and the wedding party was beautiful there on the beach with the wind blowing gently and the sunset behind them. I didn't know anyone at the wedding except for my two sons, my friend Elliot, and my ex-husband, John.

It seemed to take a long time on the beach with the photographer. When we finally went back for the reception it was night. I think I was probably the only person there with two escorts, Elliot and John. As it turned out, we were all seated at the same table. Next to us were Debby's parents, grandparents, and a couple of siblings who weren't sitting at the head table with the rest of the wedding party.

"This is cozy," Elliot said once we had sat down; but before I had a chance to respond, John had butted in to the conversation.

"Hey, if you two aren't going to drink, can I have your drink tickets?" he asked.

"Sure", I said, "knock yourself out." Elliot and I both handed over two tickets each, and John got up and immediately went to the bar. "Some things never change," I said. Elliot nodded in agreement.

The night wore on. Besides the DJ, Debby's family had hired one of her cousins, an Elvis impersonator, as part of the entertainment. He was walking around with a wireless microphone singing love songs, interrupted only by Ben, who was saying all kinds of romantic things. "This is the happiest day of my whole life," he said, and so forth.

John must have managed to acquire other drink tickets too, because he had about eight empty glasses in front of his place by the time I checked to see what had happened to him. I looked around to see where he was and spotted him coming our way with two more drinks, one in each hand. He managed to negotiate the dance floor without spilling anything and dropped down in his seat next to me. He was grinning from ear to ear.

"Hey, you probably should slow down, cowboy," I said to him,

"Hell, it's our son's wedding. I'll drink as much as I want," he said. Then he leaned closer to me and put his arm around the back of my chair. "This is some kind of circus, isn't it?" He asked.

"I must admit that Elvis is certainly a special touch," I said. He leaned closer, grabbing the table for more support; then he spoke again, only louder this time.

"If you and I had done this thing, we'd have done it right. Look at this shit will you?" He reached toward the centerpiece in the middle of the table, grabbed the bottom of the vase and pulled it towards us. The table cloth came with it and some of the dishes. "Look at this!" He said. John held up the vase for me to get a better look. "It looks like some kind of damned funeral urn." He was right about that. It was a smaller replica of the kind of urn one might see in a cemetery, except that it was painted silver and had fake ferns coming out of the top. Elvis had waltzed over to our table right about then, and he was asking Elliot what he would like to hear him sing.

"Who the f _ _ _ is that?" John asked me, and both of us started laughing. I realize now that my laughter must have encouraged him because the next thing he said got both of us kicked out, and not just from the reception, but from Ben's life too.

He sat back in his chair. At first his expression was almost angelic; then he began to laugh like the devil. His arms were crossed in front of him and he was shaking with mirth, grinning at me. He said, "Honey, these people aren't I-talian, they're just cheap Jew bastards!"

November 1999

I was still holding onto the phone. "John, are you still there?" I asked.

"I don't know much about what happened," was all he said. "But, I just wanted to tell you before Gray arrived."

"I don't know what to say."

"Well, I'm sorry." he said. There was another pause between us. "It's really hard to know what to tell you; I don't have any details except that Debby called me this morning."

"Is he still in the hospital? Can I talk to him?" I asked.

"She didn't give me that information, but I'll try to find out and get back with you," he said. "I've got to go now. We'll talk later."

That was the end of our conversation because he hung up before I could get another word in.

I felt paralyzed there on the floor next to my bedside stand. The birds were still chirping outside the window; they seemed to be my only company. I kept hearing one phrase repeating itself inside my head, only it was more like a prayer, and it was this: *Please God help me* ... I looked out the window and saw that the sky was now obscured by gray clouds. Large droplets of rain were starting to fall on the porch roof. It was as if nature were crying for me because I couldn't. I wondered then if God really knew what was going on in my life at all, or if I were really as insignificant as I felt then.

I could hear the gravel on the driveway crunching and realized that Evelyn and Micky must be home. The back door slammed, and I could hear them bringing stuff into the house. She was irritated at him again. I didn't hear what she was saying, but I could tell by her tone that he was in trouble with her. The poor kid spent most of his free time in his room downstairs, grounded for stupid infractions like not putting dishes in the dishwasher correctly or forgetting to fold her wash. It was always one thing or another.

I started down the stairs. Evelyn was shouting now. "Micky go straight to your room and don't come out again until all the clothes on the floor are folded," she said to him. They were standing in the living room, and his head was hanging down. He seemed to be inspecting the carpet on the floor. His book bag was dangling from his right arm, forming a lumpy pile on the carpet. In the other hand he held a wrinkled brown jacket. He looked more like an old hobo than an 11- year-old-boy.

"GET DOWNSTAIRS!" she screamed. Then she turned to me and with a flick of her head gestured me to follow. "Let's go," she commanded. Then she was out the door without turning to see if I had followed. I didn't have a chance to tell her I wouldn't need the ride after all. I followed her out to the driveway to explain. She was standing next to my car, lighting up another cigarette. As I approached, she blew a long stream of smoke towards the car. I remember being amazed by this because any other mere human being wouldn't have been able to light the cigarette in the first place with the rain coming down.

"I won't be needing a ride. I got in touch with the insurance agent, and it's all handled," I said. She looked at me in disbelief and then took another long drag off her cigarette.

"Do you mean I came all the way back here and you don't need the car?"

"Yeah, I was able to get the logistics sorted out, and I'm going to drive to the body shop where the rental people will meet me with a car." Her lip curled at this, and she threw the cigarette she had been smoking down on the ground. It landed near my feet and made a sizzling sound as the rain hit the lighted end. I took a step back and considered what to tell her next. I wasn't so sure she would want to hear the rest of the story.

"Look, I'm sorry you went out of your way for me. I appreciate it; I really do."

"Oh that's ok," she replied. "Everybody else takes advantage of my good nature. What makes you any different?"

"I'm not trying to take advantage of you, Evelyn," I said. It's been a rough morning, and I got some additional bad news; so it's all been kind of complex and confusing and Ben-is-in-the-hospital!" The last part of the sentence just seemed to rush out of me. I hadn't intended to tell anyone just yet, much less my newly-acquired landlady.

"What do you mean he's in the hospital?" Her surly look had transformed into one of condescension. She folded her arms across her chest now as she waited for my response. The rain was still coming down, and it was turning colder. I rubbed my hands together before holding them out in front of me, like a protective shield, as if blocking her. I felt defensive.

"He tried to kill himself; I don't know any more details than that," I blurted out. If his father calls, can you take a message for me until I get back?"

The look on her face changed to one of surprise.

She strode across the drive to where I was standing until she was so close to me I could smell the smoke on her breath. She wrapped her arms around me in a clumsy hug. I felt smothered, and the cigarette smell was nauseating. I stood awkwardly in her embrace with an intense desire to leave immediately, to be released from the hold of her arms, so sudden, so prolonged, so intense. She made me nervous.

"Let me go," I said. "I've got to get to the airport." She released me, and I went straight to my own car. Despite its outward condition, it started right up. I knew I would make it to the body shop in one piece!

As I backed down the driveway, I rolled down the window and yelled out to her. For some reason I felt sorry for her. "Don't worry; it's all going to be ok!" It was what I told all of my patients, everyone I wanted to help, no matter what was going on. Then I waved goodbye and drove down the road to the rental car facility and the airport.

Chapter 5

November 1999

Thanksgiving was clear and bright. The sky was a brilliant blue, and high up a few clouds were drifting by. I could see the entire valley from the third floor, and it looked as if it had been washed clean by the rain the day before. My car was safe in the body shop, and my younger son was still sleeping in my room. I had camped out on the floor of my studio where I had access to a coffee machine and a small refrigerator. This convenience made it possible to have breakfast without waking anyone up downstairs by being in the kitchen. I had just started on my second cup of coffee when the phone rang; I jumped up to grab it before the second ring.

This time it was Debby, my son's wife. "Hi, I guess you heard what happened," she said. "Ben is in the hospital here, and I thought that I should call because he doesn't have phone privileges yet." I was thinking to myself, *why hadn't she called me earlier*, but I held my tongue. Instead I asked, "Is Ben okay?"

"Oh yes, he was just under stress. I don't think he was sleeping much because he was getting up to feed the baby a couple times a night, and he works a lot at the restaurant," she replied. "But the baby's fine though."

She had just given birth to their child, a son, only a couple of weeks before, and I felt sorry for her having to carry so much responsibility. "It must be very difficult for you right now," I said. I knew that she didn't like me very much, especially after the incident with John at their wedding. I was hoping to use the conversation to bring us closer together.

She started to cry. "You don't have any idea how hard things have been!" she said. "He's been impossible these last weeks."

"Do you mean the baby or Ben?" I asked.

"Ben of course!" She was almost screaming into the phone now. I held the phone away from my ear and tried to imagine her standing in a phone booth in the hospital corridor, separated from her husband who was probably down the hall in the psychiatric unit. I looked out my window; the fields and hills were begging to be put on canvas. I desperately wanted to be outside in that beautiful landscape of hills when I realized that Debby was still talking to me.

"He was working all the time, and I thought he should at least help me with the baby a little bit; so he was doing the night feedings." she said. Then she started to sob again. "It's not fair, it's just not fair!" she cried.

"What's not fair, dear?" I asked.

"I can't believe he did this to me!" she said. At this point in our conversation I wasn't quite sure how to respond and still find out how my son really was without sounding unsympathetic towards her.

"I'm sorry you've had to go through so much," I said. It must be terrible, but can you tell me when can I speak with Ben?"

"I'll tell him to call you after his evaluation." she said. I could hear a great deal of commotion in the background now, and then the receiver went dead and she was gone.

Now I was faced with the situation that I hate the most, not knowing. I decided to sit around by the phone anyway, hoping that sooner or later Ben would call me. Then I would relax, I told myself.

The phone rang a few more times that morning, but it was various friends calling to wish me a happy Thanksgiving; so our conversations were short. Most of them had family dinners or parties to attend. I had already decided to take Gray out for Thanksgiving for two reasons: it gave us something to do, and I hoped it would prevent me from feeling weird and lost on another holiday. I hated holidays now. My sons were the only two family members I had left in the whole world, since the time my Mother had been locked up in the Home. I still had a brother, sister and father but none of us had talked for several years, and they were as lost to me as my Mother was. It wasn't as if we had had a fight or anything. I guess that all of us had just lost interest over the years. These things happen.

Thanksgiving vacation passed slowly. Gray and I took long walks and waited by the phone. As I look back, I think that I was numb during that time. It was almost like watching a movie. "Why do you think he did it, Mom?" Gray asked.

"Maybe the pain of being alive was too much for him." I said. "I don't know. I always thought he was happy."

Finally Ben did call, but he had kept us waiting so long that I had become anxious and afraid by then; I felt as if my heart was going to break open. Gray and I both hovered over the phone to hear what he was saying. The hospital had done some tests, he told us. They had found something in his brain that they thought had contributed to the seizures.

"What kind of seizures?" I asked.

"I was having some kind of strange day dream." he explained. "The devil was speaking to me from the mirror in my bedroom. It's happened before, but when I started to get up at night, I would see him there all the time. Then I started to see him at work, and he was talking to me, telling me stuff."

"What did he tell you?" I asked.

"Well, he told me to hurt the baby. He told me I should suffocate the baby, and that I should . . ." He stopped talking and started to sob. "I'm so sorry, he said, I didn't mean it, I didn't. I told the Doctor that I don't think I did anything to hurt him."

"I'm sure you didn't do anything like that," I told him.

"Listen, I've got to go Mom. They only allow me so long to use the phone, I'll call you tomorrow. I think they're going to keep me here for a while."

"I love you," I said.

"Me too," he said. And then we hung up. I still couldn't cry, though. I thought I should have. I thought how strange it was that I couldn't feel any of the pain the others were feeling.

The day after the holiday was cold. The wind had blown what was left of the leaves from the driveway and the lawn. Our house had been built into a great hill, and the expansive lawn was a vibrant green. A series of flagstone steps curved up through the gardens in front, and flagstone terraces had been built across the lawn, probably to keep the hill from washing away.

Gray had decided to watch a football game on TV and had settled into a big leather chair in the den, leaving me to cast about for something to do. I stared down at the lawn, watching how the last of the leaves were being caught in the dead plants that hadn't been dug up from the garden. The wind had made them come alive, moving them about in the naked branches. Meanwhile I had a good view of the road that went by the house. Cars were whizzing south along the old route traveling toward the city of Baltimore. I wondered what the people in the cars would be doing when they got to wherever it was they were going. I felt alone and lost again.

Finally I decided it was too beautiful a day to remain inside especially after all the rain we had been having recently. Another walk would do me some good. I found my leather jacket and an old hat in the back entrance of the house, and I pulled my hiking boots on, ready to go on a long jaunt. I was reminding myself that this was why I had moved into the country in the first place, and besides, walking was a good way to alleviate depression. I pulled my sunglasses on and headed out the door into the back driveway. I heard a crunch of tires on the loose gravel before I saw the old station wagon pulling up. In fact, I nearly walked into the car because my eyes hadn't adjusted to the light yet.

It turned out to be my neighbor Lewis, who lived up the road not far from us. He often came to visit, unannounced, and I gave a long sigh. I was never very glad to see him. For some reason he liked to bring us strange shaped stones and pieces of wood that he found around the reservoir. He would tell Evelyn and me that we could use all these interesting things as decoration in the gardens. Actually, I used the wood for kindling in the fireplace. Evelyn had put the stones carefully along the driveway in the back as a kind of barrier, keeping people from parking their cars on the lawn.

Evelyn and I had lots of visitors that fall, and for some reason when they drove up the back driveway they always parked on the lawn. I found out later that we had become a kind of roadside attraction for all the single males who lived in the surrounding countryside. Evelyn and I were known as the two artists who lived in the old Inn up the hill. Lewis was no exception; only he came around nearly every day.

The old station wagon pulled to an abrupt halt on the gravel. I pushed my sunglasses back on my head so that I could see better. Lewis remained in the car, rolling the window down. "Hi, how'd ya like some company?" he asked.

Truth was I really didn't want company, and the last thing I needed was Lewis tagging along on my walk. I tried to think of a good reason to send him packing when I realized that there was someone else in the car with him. The other person leaned forward now, making it possible to see them both at once. Lewis's passenger was staring at me and smiling. I moved towards the car, not sure now whether to send them on their way or to invite them inside.

"This is my friend Richard," Lewis said. I didn't reply, just held up my hand in a universal greeting. Lewis must have sensed my reluctance to invite them in because he continued talking. "We've been out all morning on a hike and thought you'd like the wood we gathered." he said. I crossed my arms in front of my chest. What I didn't need was any more firewood from Lewis.

"Gee whiz, Lewis! We're in pretty good shape with wood right now. Evelyn's friend Tommy just brought us a load last Monday." I said. I turned and pointed to the side of the house where a lumpy pile of logs lay where Tommy had dumped it. I crossed my arms again and stood there waiting for Lewis to get the hint and leave. Instead, his friend Richard was opening the door and climbing out of the car. For the first time since they arrived, his friend spoke. "Then we'll be helping you stack that wood," he said. Not even waiting for a reply, he walked directly across the drive to the pile of wood and then turned around. Richard was looking intensely at me, and I shifted nervously. "That's supposing it's okay with you if I stack your wood." he said. He was still smiling.

He had certainly taken me by surprise. "Actions speak louder than words." I finally replied. I was charmed by his boldness and by the practicality of his suggestion. I took a step forward in Richard's direction; something about him was intriguing.

"Is Evelyn home?" Lewis asked.

Already, I had forgotten Lewis. I turned back around to the car and saw that he was still sitting there. "She's in New Jersey, won't be home till sometime this evening. I said. Why don't you go inside and watch the football game with my son Gray?" Meanwhile Richard was already stacking the wood, paying no attention to me or Lewis at all. *A man of action, I thought.* How refreshing. I found I was smiling too. I felt uplifted for the first time in two days.

"C'mon Lewis; I'll show you where Gray is, and you can help yourself to whatever you want to eat," I said. We went into the house together.

"Got any beer?" he asked.

Two days latter I drove Gray back to the airport. We arrived early, and I decided to wait with him until the plane docked at the gate. All around us, groups of people were saying goodbye. Babies in strollers, young men and women in uniforms, college kids with book bags, and grandmas and grandpas were embracing, kissing one another. In that respect, we were like the rest of the crowd. Gray was leaving too.

It was then that I started to feel a pain in my chest. It swelled up and moved to my throat, one big lump. I couldn't swallow, and I couldn't talk. It was as if all the things I had wanted to say and never said, had formed a huge ball in my throat and remained stuck there. Gray patted me on the back. My suffering had arrived at the worst of times, here at the airport, in front of people I didn't even know.

"Are you okay?" he asked. It seemed as if that was the only question either of us had asked each other in the last several days. It was slightly humorous in a strange way that only he and I could appreciate. I smiled slightly.

"I'm not going to die if that's what you mean." I said.

"He's going to be fine," Gray said. "The doctors will find out what's in his head, and they will fix it."

"I don't trust doctors. The last time a doctor told me everything was going to go well, we ended up sticking my mother in the Home," I said. Then I started to cry again, little sobs; my shoulders kept going up and down. Gray gave me another hug, and we ambled over to the gate where they had started to load the plane.

"I'll call you soon," he said. Then he turned into the line with the rest of the passengers. I watched until he had rounded the corner, and then he was gone. I was left standing there in a room full of people, some coming and some going; but I felt more alone than I had in my whole life.

I walked slowly out to my car. There really wasn't any reason for me to rush anywhere now. Nobody was waiting for me to come home. There was no boyfriend, no husband, no parents calling; and most of my friends were out of town. Evelyn had gone off again for the weekend to spend time with her girlfriend on the shore. It was her ex-husband's turn to take Micky for the holiday. The house would be dark when I got there.

Chapter 6

December 1999

Monday was a work day, and I was relieved that I would have something to do besides listen for the phone to ring. In fact, I had taken it off the hook the night before. I didn't think that I could process any more information. I was tired, and I needed to sleep.

My first client to see that morning was Gertrude. I loved driving through the neighborhood where she and her family lived. I took the long way around, winding past the fish ponds with the fountains spraying water in the middle. Then I drove up the alley behind the houses, which was the best way to park; I wouldn't have to climb up all the steps leading up to the front. I had figured this out on my first visit, that there was an entrance in the back of the house. The dog greeted me at the back door, jumping up and knocking everything I had been carrying out of my hands, onto the floor.

"Scout, stop jumping! "the Mrs. called. She came out of the kitchen, wiping her hands on a dishtowel. She was a pretty blonde, slightly plump, and flushed from whatever she had been doing in the kitchen. "I'm so sorry," she said.

I wish people would stop saying that to me, I thought. "Oh that's all right!" I said. I felt clumsy and stupid standing there with jars of paint rolling all over the hallway. The Mrs. stooped over to help me pick everything up. Together we managed to fit all the paint jars back into the cardboard box I had been holding.

"Scout gets excited whenever anyone comes into the house," she explained. "Just tell him to get off next time. There you are, all together again. Gertrude's all ready for you; she even remembered you'd be coming!" She smiled brightly and then turned and went back to her household chores. Meanwhile, I retrieved my box and began the ascent of the stairs with Scout right behind me, sniffing my rear end.

I knocked at Gertrude's door, but before she answered, Scout had crashed through and was bouncing up to where she was sitting. The room was completely dark even though it was still morning. All the window shades had been pulled down, and the lights were turned off.

"Good Morning!" I cried. "Let's turn some lights on; I can hardly see you. And get those shades up!"

"I like it dark," she replied. "You may turn on the light by the table, but please leave the shades alone."

She wasn't dressed yet and was wearing only a nightdress. Her hair was pushed up into a little granny style nightcap, with hair sticking out from around the edges. She was holding a rosary in her hands, and a little black Bible lay open on her lap. The table to which she referred was the wobbly card table I had seen the week before. It had been moved over to the only window with a little bit of light coming in. On top of the table there was a tray with leftover food on it.

I picked up the tray to move it, but there wasn't any place to put it that didn't already have something else on top of it. I sighed and looked around the room. "Look, I'm just going to take the tray downstairs," I said. When I arrived back at the kitchen, though, the Mrs. was taking a pan of little cookies out of the oven. Other batches were already cooling on the tops of all the counters and the table. So, for the second time that day, I felt like the world's biggest idiot, standing there with the tray in my hands and no place to put it.

"Oh, dear, I'm so sorry!" she said. I'm in the middle of baking for the Museum's art auction this afternoon. Just put it on the floor, will you?"

"What about the dog?" I asked.

"What about him? She looked mystified at this.

"Won't he eat off the tray?"

"Oh it's perfectly okay; he eats off Gertrude's trays all the time," she said. I left the tray where she directed and went upstairs again. This time Gertrude had moved her wheelchair over to the wobbly card table in front of the window. She was leaning over the table and looking out from underneath the shade.

"Gotta keep an eye on em'," she explained.

"On whom?"

"There's some men been trying to get into my room! Why, they put their ladders up to my windows and try to get in!" she said. "That's why I always pull down the shades!" She sat back in the chair and her lower lip was sticking out the same way it had the day I had met her; so I knew better than to challenge her about the men, whoever they were.

I moved over to the table, sat down in the only chair in her room and pulled the shade about halfway up the window. She grimaced at the amount of light that was now streaming into her room, holding her hands over her eyes. "Jesus, Mary and Joseph!" she yelled.

I reached over and put my hand on her shoulder. "Settle down; if we don't have light, we can't see to paint!" I said.

"Will you pull it back down after we're done?" she asked.

"Of course I will, but we need to start painting now." I said. We had already spent enough time on preliminary stuff, and I thought we ought to be getting on with it. I pulled a piece of watercolor paper off the tablet I had brought along and started to squirt paint into her paint tray.

"I haven't painted for a long time," she said. "My hand hurts. I don't think I can do this today." She pulled a shawl that had been draped over the back of her wheelchair around her shoulders. "I'm cold," she added, as if for effect. I gave her the standard answer I give to everyone who has some kind of consideration about painting.

"That's wonderful," I said.

"What do you mean?" she asked, incredulously.

"I mean, that's just great about your hand and the fact that you haven't painted for the last 50 years or so and that you're cold. Fact is, none of that stuff is going to prevent you from painting with me!"

"Here's what we're going to do," I said. I took her hand then and wrapped it around the paintbrush just as you would hold a pencil. And I started to paint with her, me holding her hand, and her following my movements. It wasn't too long before she was holding the brush on her own and filling in the lines I had drawn on the paper.

"This is ok," she said. "The first time I took painting lessons, it was with the nuns from our parish; only they took us out to a field and told the class to just paint what you see."

"That's wonderful," I said.

"Is that your standard response for everything?" she asked.

"No."

"Well you always seem to say it. What else do you tell people who paint with you?" she asked.

I thought a minute about that; I didn't want her to think that I did the same thing with everyone. I just wanted her to participate with me, to begin moving again. "Usually I say that it's all good," I said.

"Hum, what other lies do you tell people in wheelchairs like me?"

"I'm not here to discuss other clients, Gertrude. Why don't you tell me something interesting about you instead?" I asked.

She stopped painting then, and folded her hands in her lap. She just stared at me for a long while before she spoke again. "I've got a secret," she said.

"What kind of secret?" I asked.

"I pray for people. I pray for people, and they get better, or their luck changes. When I was a kid, my grandfather used to bring all kinds of folk around when there was some kind of problem or something. Back then we didn't have the kind of medicine we have today."

"So you would pray for these people, and their luck would change; is that it?" I asked. She shifted around in her wheelchair and looked me straight in the eye.

"You don't believe me, do you?" she asked.

"Well, it is a little far fetched," I said. "Heck, I don't think I've prayed for anything or anyone since I was a little kid. I'm not so sure there even is a God that knows about me and my personal problems," I added.

"Do you have a problem, dear?" she asked.

"We all have problems, Gertrude," I said. "There's not a person on earth who doesn't have some kind of cross to bear. I mean, if you're alive, you've got issues." I hadn't planned on the discussion getting quite so personal on the first session together, and I felt somewhat uncomfortable about what she had just said. After all, she was just an old lady, with a touch of dementia.

She sighed. "Do you have something you need praying for?" she asked again.

"I don't discuss my personal life with my clients," I said.

"Give me a name." She reached into the pocket of her nightdress and pulled the rosary she had been holding earlier out in front of me for inspection. "I always pray, with this rosary, everyday," she said.

"Don't be silly; that's just one of those plastic things you can get at a county fair for a dime." I informed her. Now I was the one to sit back in my chair and fold my arms across my chest.

"Suit yourself," she said. She put the rosary back into her pocket. "I guess that we'll just have to busy ourselves and paint. That's what you've come here to do with me, isn't it? These painting lessons are supposed to be a glorious distraction from my otherwise mundane existence. Be honest with me."

"Well, yes, that's exactly why your son and daughter-in-law have hired me," I confessed.

"They're paying you to do this?" She looked absolutely shocked, put the paintbrush down and pushed herself away from the card table with such force that the water spilled and ran down one leg of the table. "This is worse than charity; and what's more, I didn't ask for it!" I could tell that she was insulted; so I didn't say anything, just waited.

"I'm the only one left in my family who's not dead. My grandfather, parents and even my brothers and sisters are all gone now," she said. Gertrude pulled the shawl tighter around her and turned away from me. There was a long silence. I wasn't sure that anything I could say would make a difference now; so again I waited. I was hoping something would pop into my head, and finally something did.

"How would you like a new friend?" I asked.

"Do I have a choice?" she asked.

"Not really. Your son has contracted with me for the next six months; so you're kind of stuck with me, I guess. I'm supposed to come here twice a week, Mondays and Thursdays. You can tell me all about your life, and we'll paint of course," I added quickly.

Gertrude smiled faintly now. "Why not? I'm not going anywhere, BUT if I don't end up liking you, you're not continuing. Have we got a deal?"

"I believe you have a new friend," I said. We shook hands. "I'll be back on Thursday, and we'll try some more painting. Is that okay?"

"We'll see," she said. "Now get out of here and take that dog with you!"

It was the first week of December, and some of the stores and shops I passed had put up Christmas decorations. There was a Salvation Army Santa Claus ringing a bell outside of the Wal-Mart Store where I got most of my art supplies. I looked down at the ground as I passed the man in the Santa suit because I had only a couple of dollars on me, and I needed them more than Santa did. Once inside the store, I was bombarded by a Christmas extravaganza.

Boxes of lights were piled up in the front, and a whole section of the flower department had been converted into a labyrinth of various sizes of Christmas trees, mechanical angels, and tinsel. I managed to find a large bottle of white tempera paint in the midst of all the decorations and got out of Wal-Mart without buying anything else, not even a single bulb.

My next stop was a private nursing home on Falls Road where I worked with an Alzheimer's unit on Monday afternoons. I unpacked the art supplies from my car and piled them on to my luggage carrier, wheeling the whole load into the long term care facility. I had just signed in at the front desk when I was met by the activities director. She surprised me. "What the hell are you doing here"? she asked me.

"This is the day that I am scheduled to work here; you know that." I replied. She put her hands on her hips then and looked me up and down. "Frankly I thought you'd be on a plane headed for Florida by now," she said.

I really wasn't in any kind of mood to discuss my son that morning because I had done nothing except answer people's questions about the whole situation for over a week now. "Drop it, Sue," I said. "He's going to be okay, and it's all under control. He's still at the hospital!"

"If it were my kid, I would have been on a plane by now," she said.

"You're making me late for the group. Besides, it's not your kid," I said.

"Have it your way!" Sue threw her hands up over her head and flounced down the hallway in front of me. "I just don't understand you, that's all."

"Well, it's easy to understand," I said, "I work because I need the money!" The double doors loomed in front of us. Sue reached them first and punched in the code. We waited together silently as they opened up into the Alzheimer's ward. I signed in again at the nurses' station before proceeding to the activity room, and at this point Sue left me. "Good luck," she said. "You'll need it." I wasn't sure if she meant about the residents or my son, but she had hurried off before I could ask her.

Already I could hear screaming and yelling coming from the activity room. Two of the residents were splayed up against the window looking out, making it difficult to get into the room. I banged on the door, hoping to catch an aide's attention. If there was a nurse around, she certainly wasn't in sight. In fact, nobody else was in sight. I pushed against the doors; and the two residents, Marge and Carl, backed off enough for me to get a foot in the door so I could force my way through.

And there they all were, either wandering around aimlessly or sitting in chairs. Most looked blankly off into space. Gardner was in his usual spot. He liked to sit in the corner by the piano with his hand down his pants. He holds a Ph.D. in philosophy; it's hard to believe sometimes. My personal favorite, Jerry came up to greet me. He was holding a belt in his hand. "I don't know where this goes," he told me. I ignored him.

One of the activity assistants had already set up the tables at the far end of the room. They had been pushed together, and newspaper was spread out on top. One resident named Kate had started picking up some of the newspaper and was folding it into little squares. Golly, I thought to myself, it's going to be one of those days!

"Come on everybody," I yelled, "Let's sit down at the table."

I rolled a length of paper out along the table and began getting out brushes. Right then the doors burst open, and in rushed Kelly, the new activity assistant. She looked flustered, but I needed her in the room with me to manage all these people; and I was relieved to see her. One by one she took them by the arm and led them over to the table where we would be painting. I had sketched out a large Christmas tree with lots of presents at the bottom; it was large and simple. Patiently Kelly placed a brush in each of their hands while I outlined the areas I wanted them to paint in.

The paint is poured into plastic drinking cups because it's easier to use and clean up afterwards, but it can also be confusing for some people who might be thirsty. Today was no exception. "Carl is drinking the red paint," Kelly said. I turned around to see how much paint Carl had managed to swallow; he gave me a big grin, causing the paint to run down both sides of his mouth. "He looks like a vampire," I said, and we both laughed.

"Who's gonna report to the nursing station?" I asked, "and who's gonna clean him up?" I use non-toxic tempera paint because dementia patients will sometimes drink anything they can get their hands on, and it's hard to watch eight residents all at the same time. "I'll fill out a report later," Kelly said, "and I'll clean him up too; you just get the others started."

I turned back to the table. They were all seated now: Marge, the housewife, Jerry, who used to be a journalist, Kate, the diva, Granville, a CPA, George, the little retarded guy, and finally Mr. Bill who swore up and down that he was a horse trainer at Pimlico Racetrack. No one knew if he had really trained horses or not because his family was never around to ask. All of them must have had money at some time or another though, or a wealthy family member, because they were being housed at the most expensive facility in town. I found out that it cost over six thousand dollars a month to keep them there, and all of them were private pays.

And now here they were, ready and waiting to paint a stupid Christmas tree with me, as if they could remember what Christmas was anyway. So, I outlined each present carefully on one end of the paper and the tree at the other end and hoped they would paint inside the lines today. I figured I could always fill in later any details that would be lost. Kelly had got Carl back to the table, and he was painting his name along the edge. His mouth had only faint pink marks now, and he was smiling.

"Hey Kelly, you can give Carl marks for active participation today; he's writing his name," I said.

"Yeah, but what about Granville?" she asked. Granville was sitting up straight in his chair, but he had been poised with a brush full of green paint, not doing anything for over ten minutes and I wasn't sure how to answer that.

"Granville, what are you doing?" I asked. He looked up at me and frowned. "It's got to be done correctly," he answered.

"Just paint the tree, kiddo."

"They're making too many people," Granville said.

"Your mother wants one for her purse," Marge replied.

Strangely enough, working with them helped me forget my own troubles; it wasn't because I felt sorry for them, either. They were just really funny.

"We are sitting here with all the children for lunch," Marge said.

They were all starting to talk randomly; so I decided on a different tactic to bring them back into reality with me and Kelly.

"Do you all want to hear the story about the time I painted with my mother?" I asked. The whole painting team looked up expectantly. They usually loved to hear this story, which I repeated nearly every time I was there. I think that they enjoyed this particular story because it made sense to them; they knew me, and now they knew my mother. I just kept reminding them that they knew.

"Your mother wants to hear it," Marge said.

"Well did you know that my Mom is in a nursing home?" I asked. They shook their heads up and down.

"Your Mom is sick?" Jerry asked.

"Yes, dear, she can't walk or talk anymore."

"It's a damned shame," he said. Then he put his head down in his hands, and he wouldn't look up. I wasn't sure if he was crying or not.

"Carl's drinking the paint again!" Kelly said.

"Well at least it's the same color; you might not have to report it twice," I said. She got up and marched Carl into the bathroom once again. The group was still shifting around at the table. The painting had been quite forgotten.

Kate had begun to gather up all the newspaper. She had gotten up from her chair and was circling the table like an orbiting planet. "There's too many pieces," she said.

"Sit down, Kate; you want to hear the story," I commanded, and she sat down. I went over to Jerry then and pried his hands from his face.

"Jerry dear, don't you want to hear the painting story?" I stood behind him and put my hands on his shoulders. I wanted to make sure that he was not upset.

"Oh yes, yes, is everyone in place for the meeting now?" he asked.

"Yes, we're all in place," I said. When I felt that I had all of their attention, I began again.

"So, I drove my Mom out into the field in my Dad's old rusty Land Rover. The sun was bright, and the wind was blowing. It was a beautiful fall day. I got out the water bottle and the paint and the paper and the brushes too."

"Do you have horses?" Mr. Bill asked.

"No, Bill shut up," I said. "You're interrupting the story."

I started again. "I got my Mom all ready to paint, and she looked at her watch and she said, 'It's twelve o'clock.' And I said, 'So what; we're here to paint.' She told me that she always has lunch at twelve o'clock and I told her that she's not having lunch today she's painting instead. Then she started to cry. You know that I want my Mom to be happy; so I packed everything back into the car."

"The table too?" Bill asked.

"Yes Bill, even the table. Then I drove out of the field and took her to get lunch. And after she had eaten lunch, I drove her back again so we could paint together."

"What about the table?" Bill asked.

"I told you Bill, even the table. So, I got everything set up again and I got my Mom positioned just right so that the sun wouldn't be in her eyes and guess what she did?" I had all of their attention now. Even Marge was leaning forward in her chair.

"She looked at her watch," I said.

"What time is it?" Kate asked.

"It was twelve o'clock again," I said. "My Mom always thinks it's twelve o'clock."

"Did she eat lunch?" Granville asks.

"No, this time she told me that she had to go to the bathroom."
This brought laughter from the group because they could all relate
to having to go to the bathroom. Jerry was laughing so much that
he dropped his paint brush, and it fell into his lap. The brush had
green paint on it, and now his crotch was green too. I hailed Kelly
for the third time in an hour.

"Oh, Kelly, we've got another accident over here." Twisting her
engagement ring, she bustled around the table to where Jerry was
sitting. "When I get married to Norman, he said I didn't have to
work anymore," she said.

"Well that's nice, dear. In the meantime, can you manage to get
him cleaned up?" I asked.

I walked over to the table again and once more got paint brushes
into everyone's hands. We started to paint again. Miraculously,
they all stayed focused for the next 30 minutes or so, and we had
what almost looked like a realistic version of a Christmas tree.

Their families will be happy, I thought. All the families like to think
that their relatives are busy doing things, as opposed to sitting in
the hallways staring at the walls, Alzheimer's disease or not.

I looked up at the clock. The hour was up. "And now it's time to
clean up, gang!" I said happily. Kelly came back again from the
bathroom; only now she had remnants of green paint on her
blouse. "I hate this job, but I need the money until I get married,"
she said. "Why do you keep coming back?" she asked me.

"I guess I love what I do," I said.

"I think you're crazy," Kelly said.

"Yeah, you're probably right, but at least I'm in the right place, am I not?"

Kelly looked vague. "Yeah, I guess," she said. "But I'm getting out of here when I marry Norman".

"Just don't forget to write in their charts about the paint," I said. I began to pack up my stuff and piled it back on my luggage carrier; I then turned to address the room at large. My dear students were all wandering off now; it was as if I hadn't even been there at all, save for the Christmas tree I had left behind.

"See you next week," I said; but nobody noticed.

I hurried out. Fortunately I managed to avoid Sue on the way out of the building. She was in a meeting and only looked up briefly as I made my way down the hallway and out the doors. I opened the trunk of my rental car and was putting the art supplies in when my cell phone started to ring. I looked down at the display, and it said *out of state,* which meant that it was someone calling from either Texas or Florida. A chill went up my spine. I answered the phone, and my son Ben was calling. I didn't even get a chance to say hello; he started to talk immediately.

"Mom, they won't let me go home; they've moved me to another place, and in 24 hours I won't have anywhere to go to." He started to cry.

"Wait a minute. What's happened?"

I realized I was almost yelling. He stopped crying long enough to tell me that Debby had called Social Services in Collier County claiming that he had tried to hurt the baby. There had been a court order issued, stating that he couldn't go home. Ben had nowhere else to go, was going to be released in 24 hours, would be out on the street by this time tomorrow. I thought about what Sue had said just an hour ago. . . "*if it were my kid, I'd be on a plane by now.*"

"Where are you being held now?" I asked. He told me the name and fortunately gave me the phone number. Hastily I wrote it all down on the back of my hand with a permanent marker pen, which was the only thing I had in my pocket. Ben was sobbing again.

"Where am I going to go? What am I going to do?" he cried.

"I'm coming down to get you," I said.

"You don't even know where the place is," he lamented.

"Don't worry, I'll find you," I said. "But I have to hang up now; I've got to make some flight arrangements."

"I love you, Mom."

"I love you too, son."

I climbed into the car and turned on the engine. Meanwhile I started to call the next nursing facility I was supposed to visit that afternoon to cancel the class. Then I proceeded to call all the places I would have been visiting the next day and managed to cancel everything else too. Fortunately, everyone was very sympathetic. "Take the whole week off," one activity director told me. "Unfortunately, I can't. I need the money," I said. I drove the whole way home planning how I would get to Florida and wondering if I even had enough left on my credit card to charge the plane fare. One thing was certain; I was going to be cutting it close.

'Twas grace that taught my heart to fear, and grace my fears relieved. How precious did that grace appear, the hour I first believed."

Rev. John Newton

Chapter 7

December 1999

It was very early in the morning, and I was driving my rental car down Falls Road towards the airport. In spite of not getting much sleep the night before, I felt more awake and alive than I could remember feeling in a long time. Maybe it was because I was finally able to do something about my son Ben, or maybe it was just plain ordinary fear. This was a time in my life when I was having trouble telling the difference between fear and excitement. Either way, it seemed that not knowing the difference was in my favor today. I looked down at my watch for the hundredth time. It was 5am.

I did the math in my head again. My plane left for Florida at 7am, making one stop at Dulles airport and then finally arriving in Ft. Meyers at 2:18pm. I had to pick up a rental car and drive an hour from the airport to where my son was being held, which would take me up to 3:30pm if all went without a hitch. The problem was that the last plane that day departed at 4:53pm. It left me with virtually no time to catch that last flight and return a rental car.

I couldn't spend the night in Florida because I didn't have enough money left over after purchasing the plane tickets. I was broke, and my VISA card had reached its limit. If I didn't get out on the last flight, I would be spending the night on the streets of Naples with my son. Evelyn had given me sixty-eight dollars that she was planning to use to buy Micky new sneakers. She had gotten up to see me off that morning.

"Here, take this money with you," she told me. "It's all the cash I've got on me, but you might need it for something. I think you will need it more than we do."

"Thanks," I said. It has always been difficult for me to accept anything, and I felt especially humbled this morning. I was taking her kid's sneaker money for goodness sake; but the thing was, I needed the money too. I crunched the money into my back pocket and left by the back door. Evelyn followed me out into the gravel driveway, and just before I got into the car I thanked her as best I could.

"I really appreciate this; I'll pay you back as soon as I can," I said.

"Be careful," was all she said, and then she went back into the old house.

I had called Debby the night before, after I made the flight reservations, to ask her if she could pick me up at the airport. I had explained that I didn't have enough time to pick up Ben, get back and leave on the last flight. I also explained that I didn't have enough money to spend the night anywhere.

"Can you help me?" I asked.

"No."

E. J. Cockey

"What about someone in your family?" I asked.

"We don't help people like you," was what she said.
I was stunned. Perhaps a whole minute went by before I could
speak again. "I'll remember that," I said.

"F_ _ _ you," she said, and then she hung up.

I looked down at my watch again. It was 5:10 am. The sky was
just starting to get light. Pinky orange light was coming up in the
east; dark blue clouds drifted along close to the horizon. I could
just barely make out the outline of the city. *I'm coming, Bubba! I'm
coming to get you!* was the only thing running through my head.

It had taken exactly 43 minutes to drive to the airport. I knew this
because I had been looking down at my watch every minute or so.
As I swung the car into the long-term parking lot, I could see a
transport bus a couple of rows from me. The driver was waiting for
a short line of people to board. I was traveling light. I had two
empty suitcases with me and a book entitled *Surviving
Schizophrenia* The suitcases would be used to pack whatever
Ben had managed to salvage of his belongings. My money, credit
card, and driver's license, were all crammed in the back pocket of
my jeans.

I jumped out of the car, grabbed the two suitcases, and slammed
the door, all the time keeping my eye on the bus. It hadn't taken
off yet, and I ran towards it, waving one arm in the air. "Wait for
me; wait!" I yelled. I ran desperately towards the open door and
was able to climb the few steps into the relative warmth inside.

Two rows of people already seated looked up at me as the bus
took off. There was standing room only, and I grabbed onto a
hand grip that hung from a bar in the bus. *"I'm coming, Bubba. I'm
coming."*

The bus dropped me off in front of the terminal where there was a baggage check for United Air. I didn't have any bags to check; so the entry process was expedited, and I got a boarding pass outside the terminal. I entered by the automatic doors and went directly to a panel of electronic data on the wall. The panel was a constant stream of information updating arrival and departure times for travelers. My flight was scheduled to leave at 6:58 am, which gave me almost an hour to find the gate and sit down.

This I accomplished easily; but when I finally sat down, the seriousness of my situation was overwhelming. The excitement of leaving and driving to the airport had now transformed into fear. I was having a hard time breathing. Thinking about the possibility of having to spend the night in a strange city had left me breathless. I looked at my watch again. It was 6:15 am, and I was wondering whom I could call to assure me that this was the right thing to do, when Gertrude came to mind.

It was a silly notion actually. I had just met the old woman; she didn't even know me or my situation. What was I going to say? "Hi, this is your art teacher, and I need some advice?" *She's going to think you are out of your mind!* But I remembered what she had told me the day before.

"I pray for people," she had said. "I pray for people, and they get better."

I knew that she had her own phone, and I also knew her number. On the opposite wall from where I sat, there were two pay phones, and nobody was using either one. I had nothing to lose, actually, nothing in the world. I had already sold everything worth anything, and was down to a rental car and Mickey's shoe money. What the hell if I woke her up. She was a good Catholic and might forgive me, or she might forget my phone call within ten minutes. She had dementia. Either way, I still had nothing to lose.

I got up slowly and walked to the other side of the hallway where the two pay phones were. I dropped a quarter into the slot and dialed Gertrude's number. It rang six times before she answered. I was holding my breath and counting the rings.

"Hello?"

"Gertrude, this is your art teacher," I said. I was breathless again.

"It's who?"

"Your art teacher," I said.

"What time is it?" she asked. "I'm still in bed. Did I oversleep again?"

"No, no, it's very early Gertrude. I am calling to ask you a favor.""

"Are you coming today, dear?" She sounded so sweet, just like a wonderful fairy godmother. I could imagine her in the little bed with pink blankets covering her and the black plastic rosary on top of the covers.

"No, actually I'm at the airport, Gertrude. I'm going to Florida today to pick up my son, Ben. He's in trouble, and I need to help him."

"Oh my," Gertrude said. I could hear her shifting around now.

She was probably arranging her granny cap and taking a drink of water from the glass she kept beside her bed.

"I have a favor to ask of you," I said. She was still shifting around, and I wasn't sure if she had heard me. "Did you hear me, Gertrude?"

"Yes, dear, what is it?" she asked.

I took another gulp of air. I had sixty-eight dollars in my pocket and not enough time to get my son and come home today. What I needed was direct intervention of the supernatural kind.

"I need you to pray for me and Ben, that we'll get home tonight," I stammered.

"Why of course I will, dear. Why I'll start right now, and you have a nice day," she said; and then she hung up before I could explain anything further. *Oh, good Lord, what if she doesn't remember?* I hung up the receiver on the pay phone just in time to hear them call my flight. I would be boarding soon; I would be flying off into the void, not knowing whether I could even get back, and I was going anyway.

Maybe Kelly was right after all; I was crazy. I had just called an old woman with dementia. Worse still, maybe there was no God after all, at least not one who heard petty troubles. There wasn't time to mull this over or even cry.

The little plane held only sixteen people, and the pilot served as the flight attendant as well. "There won't be complimentary services," he told us. The plane won't be in the air long enough." I looked around. The plane was filled with businessmen going to Washington, D.C. Most had on dark suits and carried brief cases.

The only other woman sat down next to me. She was at least as old as Gertrude and carried a large brown paper bag that was filled with a shawl and her lunch. I found this out because she kept up a steady monologue during the entire flight. She also told me that she was scared to fly; and every time the plane took a dip or a turn she would gasp and grab my hand.

"Pray with me," she demanded, "so we won't be killed!"

The plane touched down at 8:15am and rolled to a complete stop. It was a puddle jumper and couldn't dock at the terminal; instead a crew of two men rolled a metal staircase out onto the airfield and right up to the door of our plane. My old lady companion started to wring her hands.

"I'm afraid of heights," she said. "What if I fall and break my leg on those awful stairs?"

"Don't worry. I'll help you," I said. So together we made it down the metal stairs, and I held her arm as we crossed the air field and went into the Dulles terminal. She was met almost immediately by a scraggly group of apparent family members who greeted her as if she were the queen of England. For a brief moment I was jealous of her. She had a family, and I was by myself.

I ambled along the concourse and found another information panel. My flight was still scheduled to leave on time for Ft. Meyers. It would be leaving Dulles at 11:45am. I had about three hours to wait for the plane, and I thought how ironic it all was. Here was a gap of three hours, and all I was asking for was 20 minutes. I had done the math again, and I was positive that if the flight took off twenty minutes early I would have just enough time to get Ben and get home. . .today.

My stomach was rumbling, but I decided not to spend any of my money, just in case I would need to feed Ben later on. Instead I sat down in front of a television and opened my book on schizophrenia. I was interested in the weather forecast for Ft. Meyers and Naples, hoping for sunshine and not rain. I didn't think I would be able to take it if we had to walk around the city all night long in the rain. It had never occurred to me to bring an umbrella.

I opened the book and started to read, intermittently watching the weather channel. I don't know how long I sat there, but after a while a man came up to me. He was dressed in a tan uniform with a United Air patch on his sleeve. A plastic name badge hung around his neck.

"I have never seen anyone read and watch T.V. at the same time before." he said, in a lilting Indian accent. I looked up from my book.

"Are you talking to me?" I asked.

"Yes, Miss," he said, and then he added, "Are you all right?" He had an inquisitive look on his face. My first impulse was to tell him I was fine and to move along. I closed my book, gathered my empty bags, and stood up. We were face to face now. He hadn't moved an inch. "I'm fine," I said, and then I sat back down and opened up the book again, indicating that our conversation was over.

"Are you a therapist or something?" he asked.

"Why would you think that?" I asked.

"In my opinion schizophrenia isn't necessarily a topic any normal person would read unless they were a therapist or something like that," he said.

I thought, *what's it going to take to get rid of this guy?* I can't remember why I decided to tell him the reason I was going to Florida. Maybe it was only because he was somebody to talk to, and I was afraid and alone. At any rate, I told him all about Ben and why I had to bring him back to Baltimore.

"Gee," he said, "I bet you could really use a cigarette."

"Yeah, right, but we're in Dulles airport, and there's a no smoking rule," I said.

He patted his badge knowingly. "True for most, but I work for United Airlines, and we've got an area where the pilots and flight attendants can smoke," he said. "Interested?" I looked down at my watch to check the time. There was still over an hour before my flight left.

"Oh my, yes," I told him.

"Then follow me."

I normally don't follow strangers, but I had already embarked on a wild enough adventure to rescue Ben. I followed him. He led me back to the gate area, and we walked down one of the boarding ramps. Instead of getting on a plane, though, we went down another metal staircase that led out to the field. Then we walked around the side of the building where there was a yard fenced in with wire. It formed a kind of cage. There were several pilots and flight attendants standing around an old oil drum, smoking cigarettes.

The scene had an end-of-the-world quality about it because the whole enclosure was rusted and dilapidated. As I got closer I could see that the oil drum had been filled with dirt and that that was where they were throwing their butts. In contrast to the wire cage, the pilots looked brand new and crisp in their navy blue uniforms and white hats. My companion said hello to a couple of them and then threw his arm around me in a familial gesture indicating that I had clearance. He reached into his pocket and pulled out a pack of Cool Filter Kings and handed a cigarette to me. It wasn't my brand, but I gratefully took it anyway.

"This is wonderful," I said. I was beginning to think that Gertrude must be praying for me by now. After all it looked as if I had been granted a smoke break from the Almighty.

My new friend finished his cigarette and threw it into the oil drum. "Good luck with your son," he said. I must get back to work; but if there is anything else I can do, let me know."

I laughed at this. His offer seemed like a wry joke. "What is so funny?" he asked. He looked perplexed now.

"Listen, what I need you can't give me," I said.

"And that is?"

"I need to land in Fort Meyers twenty minutes early so that there is enough time to pick up my son, then get back to the airport and come home, all in the same day. I'm sort of flying on a wing and a prayer," I said.

He smiled "Then today is your lucky day." He pulled a radio phone from his belt and began talking to someone. I was still baffled.

"What do you mean?" I asked. He put the phone back onto his belt and began talking, but I couldn't hear anything he was saying. It was a windy day, and a large jet was taxiing up the field toward us. The roar of the engines drowned out everything he was saying. I stepped closer. "I can't hear you!" I yelled.

He didn't answer; instead he just motioned for me to follow him. He was heading back to the terminal, so I trotted along behind. I glanced down at my watch; it was 11:05 am. We went into a side door, and I realized that we had arrived at my gate. The waiting area was jammed with people, and the sign was lit up in red for Ft. Meyers. Many were already standing in a line waiting to get boarding passes.

He stopped and pulled out his phone, but I couldn't hear what he was saying again. My ears were still ringing from the jet engines out on the field. He finally got off the phone and turned back towards me. "Your flight is leaving early; you better get going." he said. I was incredulous. I heard what he said, but I felt as if my feet were cemented to the floor. I couldn't move.

"What do you mean? How can it leave early?" I asked. His smile was so broad this time I could see all of his teeth. *Oh my God, I have been following a crazy person around the airport,* I thought. *I'm going to have to start screaming for a security guard.* But he went on to explain.

"I'm in charge of scheduling outbound flights for United Air," he said. "And you will be landing in Fort Meyers at two o' clock."

"What about the other passengers?" I asked. He held up the radio phone for me to see.

"I've been in communication with the flight attendant over there." He waved his hand in the direction of the desk where the attendant was handing out boarding passes. "Everyone's either here or accounted for, and if I were you, I'd get in line. United Air flight 547 will be leaving soon."

"I don't know what to say! How can I thank you?" I asked.

"Just take care of your son, and God bless you both," he said. We shook hands, and I turned to get in line with the other passengers. It didn't even occur to me until I was in the air that a miracle had just happened.

For the first time in over a week, I knew that Ben was going to be okay.

Chapter 8

December 1999

The next day, Ben and I got up early. The sun was out, but there was a chill in the air. It was probably around 50 degrees; yet it seemed as if it should be warmer, even though it was early December. The grass on the front lawn was a brilliant green, and Ben had gone outside to breathe in the fresh air. He had borrowed one of my large sweaters to wear; most of his winter clothes had remained behind in Florida. I looked out the window from the kitchen to make sure he wasn't going to wander off. Frankly, it made me nervous to see him out on the lawn. Now that we had made it back to Baltimore, I didn't want to lose him.

He had been emotional on the way home and seemed disoriented. I hadn't been prepared for that. Fortunately, though, United Air had served a hearty snack on the return flight, and I had used some of Micky's sneaker money to purchase us both a beer once we had gotten our seats on the plane. The beer calmed us, and Ben had slept.

Now it was Wednesday morning, and Evelyn had driven Micky to school; so Ben and I had the kitchen to ourselves for the time being. My plan was to take him to the emergency room at the hospital, since he was no longer under the care of a doctor. It was the only way to have him evaluated. Under the circumstances I didn't know whether he was going to need a psychiatrist or a neurosurgeon.

There wasn't much in the refrigerator to fix for breakfast. There never seemed to be anything to eat, in spite of the fact that I went grocery shopping all the time. It was one of those roommate details that Evelyn and I hadn't worked out yet, and I was beginning to develop a resentment about it, especially this morning. I decided to speak with her about it some other time. Sixty of Micky's sneaker dollars still remained in my possession.

I made toast and coffee, and we got ourselves together in no time at all. Before I knew it, we were in the car, back on the same route I had taken the day before, driving south into Baltimore. I reasoned that if we got to the hospital early enough, we wouldn't have to wait as long.

Wrong. A very obese nurse brought us into a small room to do what she called an 'intake'. We squeezed in with her, but because of her immense size it felt more like a broom closet than a room. Her main concern seemed to be whether or not Ben had medical insurance, what was the company's name, address, and so forth. It wasn't until these data had been established that she began to take his pulse, blood pressure and the like. After that, the interview process got a little sticky. She asked Ben the questions, and I answered them.

"Exactly why are you here today?" she said.

"He tried to commit suicide," I said. She registered no surprise about this, never looking up, writing it down in a little box on her chart.

"When and where did this suicide attempt take place?" she asked.

"Right before Thanksgiving, in . . ."

She cut me off in mid-sentence. "I believe that Ben is an adult and can answer the questions himself," she said. "Why don't you take a seat in the waiting room?"

"I am staying right here," I said, and then as an afterthought added, "You'll be needing me to fill in his medical history." At this Ben began to nod his head in agreement.

"I'm a little fuzzy," he said. I had to agree with that. Frankly we both looked a little the worse for wear. He had a day's growth of beard, and my striped sweater looked completely out of place over the gray sweat pants he had pulled on earlier that morning.

As for me, I had yanked my hair back into a ponytail and was wearing my old leather jacket with the same jeans from the day before. My hiking boots had mud on them, and one of Ben's sneakers had a hole in the toe.

The nurse looked at both of us then and must have sized up the situation because all she said was, "Suit yourselves." In the end it took us over an hour recounting the circumstances that had led us to the emergency room that morning. The nurse's manner had softened considerably. She even let me answer some of the questions. Finally she led us to another room and told Ben to go in, take off his clothes and put on a hospital gown. Then she gave me my instructions.

"There is a cafeteria on the fifth floor. Why don't you go get a cup of coffee," she said. "We'll need to take a CAT scan before we can determine anything, and it will be a while." She certainly wasn't wrong about how long it was going to take. Six hours later, Ben and I were still waiting. It was 2 o'clock in the afternoon, and I had drunk at least ten cups of coffee.

I called my best friend Elliott and asked him to come over to the hospital and bring some sandwiches. He didn't have a regular job, taught art at a local school and usually had ample time in the afternoon. I wanted him to relieve me and sit with Ben for a while. Even though I am used to being inside hospitals, it's a vastly different experience when it's your own son in there.

Elliott finally arrived 45 minutes later carrying a bag full of oranges and some candy bars. "What the hell is this crap, Elliott?" I asked. "Did you rob an old bag lady on the way here? I was thinking more along the line of a submarine sandwich and some magazines." My nerves were fried, and I was getting testy.

"Hey, take a break and get off my ass," Elliott said. "I'm doing the best I can!" He pushed me out of the room and into the hall. Suddenly we were standing in the middle of chaos; bells were ringing, and doctors and nurses were rushing from one patient to another. The place was packed with humanity and noise. Many of the patients were separated only by sheer white curtains that hung from tracks in the ceiling. "You better get your shit together," he said. "Ben needs you."

He was right of course, but I was tired and scared. We had been in the emergency room for a long time, and I had run completely out of patience. "I can't just stand around anymore!" I told him. "What am I going to do now?"

"Listen, take a walk or something. I'll stay here with Ben," he suggested.

I looked up and down the hall, hoping to catch up with the doctor who had seen Ben earlier. We were still waiting to hear about the results of the CAT scan. Not knowing anything has always been worse for me than hearing bad news. "I'm going to wander around and see what I can find out from the doctor," I told Elliott. "I'll be back soon."

"Take your time," he said. "Ben is sleeping anyway, but I'll be here if he wakes up."

I walked down the hall and turned left where earlier I had seen several doctors in white lab coats looking at x-rays on back-lit screens. That area was empty now; so I just kept following signs that read 'Special Imaging'. No one paid any attention to me; so I kept going, hoping to find somebody who could tell me something, anything.

I took another left and found myself in a brightly lit corridor where there were two men, both in white lab coats, standing and talking together a short distance away. One man had a gray beard. I could see his profile fairly well, and he looked vaguely familiar but I couldn't remember where I had seen him before. I was trying to place him when they both turned towards me and I could see the bearded man's face clearly. He was smiling. Then I remembered.

"Richard! Is that you?" We were both taken by surprise.

"What are you doing here?" he asked. He walked towards me and we shook hands. "I thought you were a college professor or something." I said. At this he threw his head back and laughed. His colleague must have thought this was very funny, because he started laughing too. Richard jotted something on a note pad "I'll talk with you about that case later." he said. His colleague turned and left. We were alone in the corridor now.

"So, what are you doing here?" he asked.

"My son had a CAT scan earlier today, we've been waiting for hours, and I thought I would try to find a doctor who could tell me what was going on," I said. I started to cry then. I didn't want to cry, but there I was, crying in the corridor. Little hiccups were coming out of my throat. I felt stupid and ashamed; I barely knew this man. Richard put his arm around my shoulders.

"Don't fret. I'm a radiologist," he said. "Let's go find those films and see what's going on."

"I thought you were a history professor," I said. He grinned.

"What ever made you think that?" he asked.

"I think it's the beard," I said.

And so he led me back down the hall, to the wall of illuminated panels. Beneath the lighted wall there was a long bench, and on the bench was a tall stack of oversized envelopes. Richard shuffled through them, and after a few moments he found what he was looking for. He pulled what looked like a large negative out of the envelope he had selected and put it up on the lighted screen. It looked like a lot of black and gray and white blobs to me. The blobs were repeated over and over again on the film. I watched his profile as he surveyed the screen. He was a handsome man, but the gray beard made him look older than he probably was. I wondered what he looked like without it, but he interrupted my thoughts.

"There are five areas in question here," he said. "They might be little bleeds or they could very well be small masses that have been there for a long time. Does your son have a history of seizures?"

"Yes. We were here about a year ago, but nothing was conclusive. I wanted him to get more tests, but he moved out of state before that could happen."

"Why?"

"It's a very long story, Richard. I'll tell you about it some other time, but the point is what should I do today?"

"I'm going to call up the film library and see what we have on file. I want to compare films and see what has changed, if anything. Then we'll determine what to do." he said. Now I interrupted him.

"He tried to kill himself," I said. Richard frowned.

"I think you'll need to tell me more," he said.

I never got the chance to tell him the story, though. Before I could relate another thing, he was paged. I understood all too well. He was a doctor and probably had a hundred patients to see that day; yet he had given me more than my fair share of time. He was one of those rare individuals who are kind to others, no matter where you meet them or what the circumstances are. On the first occasion I had met him, and even now, I felt better after being around him.

I turned to go, and he touched me on the arm. "I'll look at those films as soon as I can," he said. "Why don't you go get yourself a cup of coffee in the meantime?"

"It seems as if everyone's been telling me to drink coffee all day," I said, and then I thanked him again for taking the time to talk with me.

"It's my pleasure," he said. Then I left and went back to find Elliott and Ben. I'd been missing long enough. As I walked back to Ben's room I thought to myself, H*e's a great guy, but after today I'll probably never see him again.*

Much later the emergency room doctor gave us the report. On the basis of what Richard had seen on the CAT scan, there would be no need to operate; but he and the other doctors recommended that Ben spend some time in the psychiatric hospital for evaluation and stabilization. It was 8 pm, and we had spent the last twelve hours in the emergency room. Elliott had left earlier to teach his night class. Ben and I had received the news together.

"Can you come with me, Mom?" he asked. "I don't want to go to another hospital by myself!"

"I can't go with you this time son," I said. "But I promise to see you tomorrow after work. They are going to transport you in the ambulance. It's some kind of hospital regulation, and I can't come along." He looked down at his hands and began to cry.

"I miss my son," he said.

"I know dear; so do I."

Chapter 9

December 1999

Once Ben was institutionalized and safe for the time being, I was able to get back to work, which was a relief for me. I reasoned that if I could get back into my normal routine, life would get easier, and the crisis would soon be over.

My first client on Thursday morning was Gertrude. I was eager to see her. I wanted to talk about her prayer life, but even more, I needed to tell her about the help that had come my way. I drove down her street with the fish ponds in the middle. The fountains had been turned off for the winter. There were mallard ducks swimming in the water, and a couple of migrant workers were cleaning dead leaves out of the water. Everything seemed to be in order there, and I enjoyed the view. I wondered what it would be like to live on a street where everything was perfect. I drove around to the alley behind the Professor's house and parked my car. They had given me a key to the house. The Mrs. had told me earlier that she would be in meetings all week long and to let myself in. My other duty was to make Gertrude lunch before I left. The nurse practitioner had given explicit instructions about what lunch would consist of: a small bunch of grapes, three slices of American cheese, a bran muffin, and one cup of hot tea. There was a list waiting for me on the kitchen counter on top of a brown serving tray. I read the list while I looked around the kitchen. The Mrs. collected roosters; they were everywhere.

The dog met me halfway up the stairs to Gertrude's room. Otherwise the house was empty. I knocked on the door to her room, got no response, and knocked again. I waited with the dog in the hall. Still no answer. I pushed the door open and went in. The room was dark as a bat's cave. I couldn't see a thing until I found the light switch on the wall. Suddenly I could see. Gertrude was still in bed, and it was nearly noon.

There was a breakfast tray on the card table which had a bowl of cereal, a large glass of milk, half a banana, and a handful of assorted medications there as well. Little pink capsules, long white pills, a tiny round caplet that had been broken in half, and some clear gel caps were lying in a cup on the side of the tray.

While I was checking out her tray, the dog had managed to climb up on the side of Gertrude's bed and was licking her face. She moaned and turned over on her side, facing away from me. She had rolled towards the wall, exposing lumpy bed linens and a stack of Good Housekeeping magazines underneath a pile of blankets at the foot of her bed.

One thing was certain; she didn't look like anyone who could elicit the attention of God. I remembered that my fraternal grandmother used to tell me that God worked in mysterious ways. By the look of things, this seemed as true today as it was when my grandmother was telling me.

E. J. Cockey

I cleared my throat and walked over to where Gertrude was lying. The dog had jumped down on the floor now and was on his back, begging to have his belly rubbed. I pushed him aside with my foot; he gave a squeal and barked. The commotion woke up Gertrude, and she sat straight up. A red plastic rosary fell to the floor as she jolted upright. Suddenly we were face to face.

"What are you doing here?" she asked, rubbing her eyes.

"It's my day," I said. She looked baffled at first, and then I could see realization dawning on her face.

"Ah yes, you're my art instructor. Well, missy, I'm not painting now," she said. "You'll have to come back later today."

I felt a jab of anger. Who did she think she was, anyway? She couldn't just order me around! I had a schedule to keep. Other patients were waiting to see me too. I told her this.

"Well, change your schedule!" she said. Her jaw was jutting out as she got out of the bed. There was a disgusted look on her face.

"Don't just stand there; get my walker!" At that point it seemed easier to get the walker than to argue. I complied.

"Where are you going?" I asked.

"To use the facilities. Now get out of my way!" she cried. And with that, she wheeled her way to the door and to the bathroom down the hall. I was left with the dog, who had come over to sit by my side. He seemed to be grinning up at me.

While I waited for Gertrude I surveyed her room. Her dresser had most of the drawers pulled out, and there was a wild variety of materials, clothes, books and boxes inside. I edged my way over to get a better view of the contents, hoping that she would take a while in the bathroom and not catch me looking through her stuff. There was a pile of stockings that had been tied into knots in one drawer, and underneath was an old photo album. It was made out of red leather that looked as if it had been opened thousands of times. The leather was cracked and worn.

Gingerly I pulled the red album out from under the stockings and opened it. Inside the pages were crumbling. There were only a few photos; they were all black and white and had faded. I looked at one of a pretty little girl with dark hair. She had on a white dress and was squinting. On the back of the photograph it said *1947, Jean's first communion*. I guessed that the little girl must be Gertrude's daughter, judging from the date. I shuffled through the album, looking for other pictures from her past. Two others especially caught my attention: one was a wallet sized wedding photo, and the other was of a much younger Gertrude with a fancy hat, standing in front of a white porch. It might have been Easter time because there were some little flowers coming up. Gertrude was holding a purse, and all ready to go to church.

I was pleased that all the images I had uncovered so far suggested she had lived a happy life, but suddenly I was startled back into the present. I could hear her footsteps coming back down the hall and the scraping of her walker as she pushed it over the carpet. I shoved the red album back under the stockings and made certain that it all looked as I had found it, then stepped back from the dresser just as she banged her way into the room.

"Help me, don't just stand there!" she yelled. Quickly I walked over to the door and opened it for her. I felt guilty after snooping through her stuff. She came into the room and went directly over to the card table where the breakfast tray was, sat down, and started to pour milk on the cereal. There was a folding chair on one side of the table; so I sat down too because I didn't know what else to do.

Gertrude reached over and patted my hand. "Don't worry, child. I really don't care if we paint at all." Then she cut the banana into little pieces. "I haven't had my breakfast yet," she told me, as if that would explain everything.

I glanced over at the clock in her room; it said 1:09 pm. It was a large digital clock that had bright red numbers which anyone could see clearly from the other end of a football field. *I had another twenty minutes before I had to leave, and we hadn't painted a thing.*

"Let's paint a basket," I said suddenly.

"You want to do magic?" she asked.

I rolled my eyes at this remark before I realized that she probably couldn't hear me. I tried again.

"Let's paint instead!" I was almost yelling now.

"You want me to go to bed?" she asked.

"Never mind, just eat your cereal," I said.

"Thank you dear. I'll just finish my breakfast," she said. Gertrude sat back in her chair and smiled graciously at me. She looked angelic, not like the old lady who had just messed with me for lack of anything better to do.

She continued to eat her cereal as I had suggested, and we didn't paint anything that day. I left early, not caring if her family liked it or not. She didn't pay any attention to me until I was almost out her door. I already had my hand on the doorknob to her room when she spoke again.

"Oh, missy," she smiled sweetly now, "I have a bit of advice to impart."

I turned around, the better to hear what Gertrude was going to tell me. She held up her spoon, filled with bran cereal and spilling over with milk. The milk was dribbling on her bathrobe, but she didn't seem to notice. Instead, her eyes were fixed on me. The dog sat beside her, and I swear that he was still grinning at me. I waited by the door, my anticipation heightened by the long pause.

"Live and learn," she said.

I closed her door with a sigh and quietly descended the stairs.

My next stop was the hospital. I took my time getting there. The traffic was relatively calm at this time of day, and I didn't feel that I had to rush. I felt I had all the time in the world because I had left Gertrude's house earlier than expected, gaining an additional five minutes by the time I pulled into the hospital's parking lot. For some reason or another, five minutes seemed like a lot of time to spend with myself. I sat in the car, letting the engine run, feeling the hot air coming through the vents under the dash. It felt warm, wonderful and good, but I was morose.

I looked up to the second floor where Park Unit was. Already there were several of my patients looking out the front windows and waving at me. I was tired, but I couldn't tell them that, could I? My life had suddenly taken a radical turn for the worse, in every possible way, and I felt orphaned and alone in the world.

The problem was I couldn't share any of my feelings. For one thing, I needed to be strong for Ben, and for another, I didn't trust anyone else.

It seemed that it always had been this way and that it always would be this way. I always ended up having to go though crises by myself. I started thinking how unfair life had been to me. *Poor me.*

Already the sun was getting lower in the sky, and there was a chill in the air. On the western side of the street there was a pale orange glow near the horizon. In front of the hospital there were several men hanging tiny white lights in the trees, which they had turned on. The strings of lights looked surrealistic spread out all over the lawn, while the men were small elfin men, in brown uniforms, bending over all the lights. I looked at my watch; my five minutes were up. I got out of the warm car and walked into the hospital.

Inside the front lobby the entire activity staff was busy pulling green pine boughs from numerous boxes that were scattered all over the floor. *I'll Be Home for Christmas* was playing on a portable radio, and the atmosphere was very upbeat and jolly. The activities cart was parked off to one side of the lobby, filled with large containers of paint. Alex saw me first and jumped up from where he had been unwrapping a bundle of Christmas tree lights.

"They're all ready for you upstairs," he said. "I'll be along in a minute."

"See ya up there," I said. I pushed the cart in front of me and got into the elevator to go up to Park Unit. There seemed to be tinsel everywhere, but it only made me feel more depressed. Once I got off on the second floor, I could hear children singing all the way down the hall. Their voices sounded high pitched and bright, and they were slightly off key. I waited patiently for them to finish. Standing behind the tables that had already been set up, their teacher must have known that I was next on the activity agenda because as soon as she saw me, she stopped playing and began to gather her singers into a tight little group. The children began to put on their coats. I felt as if I should say something nice to her, since none of the activity personnel were around to wrap things up.

"Good show," I said, thinking to myself how pitiful they really were.

She looked me straight in the eyes, as if she already knew I couldn't care less, and folded her hands in front of her. "Thank you. We've been practicing for weeks," she said.

Now I felt worse. I had managed to insult little children and their teacher with my attitude alone. I was mulling this over when suddenly someone grabbed my shoulder.

"What's up, girl?" said a cheerful voice. It was Alex. He was wearing a red Santa hat, and he was smiling from ear to ear. Before I could say anything, he had walked past me and was starting to gather everyone together around the tables. There were at least twenty people or so left over from the singing assembly, and Alex was moving them all into place.

"Sister Marie was wondering if they could paint a Christmas mural today," Alex said.

"What kind of Christmas mural?" I asked. "The manger scene, a Christmas tree or do we have to do something politically correct?"

"Go the religious route; this is a Catholic hospital, remember?" he replied.

"Whatever you want; I'm your trusted servant," I said and bowed.

"You're such an asshole," I heard someone say. I looked down at the people parked around the tables in their wheelchairs. Betty was the closest and she was looking over at Mary across the table.

"I said, you're a real asshole," she said again.

"Screw you too," Mary said back. I didn't feel like breaking up an argument, but I walked over behind Betty and put both of my hands on her shoulders.

"Wassa matter wi' you?" she asked, looking up at me.

"My oldest kid is sick," I told her.

"My husband just up and died two year ago. I kinda hate this time o' year too," she said. Then she reached out and put her one good hand on my arm.

"The Lord giveth and the Lord taketh away," she said.

The poignancy of her words caught me off guard. She had touched upon my deeper fear: my son could die. Nervously, I started to laugh, and then she began to laugh too. "You've really cheered me up this time," I said.

"What's so funny? Are you laughing at me?" Mary asked. Betty leaned forward in her chair. She pulled her stick out from under the blanket on her lap and shook it at Mary.

"I'm gonna knock yo' silly head off," she threatened. "Her chile is sick."

"That's enough out of both of you," I told them. "Let's not fight. I'm here to paint the manger scene. Are you going to help with this project or continue to argue?"

"Let's paint!" Betty yelled.

"My head hurts," Mary cried.

"Just shut up and paint, Mary. I'm really not in the mood today for your whining, okay?"

She looked down at her hands.

"I don't want to paint today," she said.

"Fine," I said. "That's just fine."

My next stop was the mental hospital where Ben was. The hospital was on my way home, and I was making my first attempt to visit him. It was already nightfall, and the sky was dark blue. I could see the lighted windows in the hospital and wondered which room was his. I knew Ben was in one of the locked-down units, but I didn't know where to go. I pulled into the lot closest to the road and looked around again. There was a sign that said Administration and another that pointed to Adult Residential. I decided to go in on the residential side and got directions from a young girl who was working the front desk. She was very positive and happy, and I resented her immediately.

I walked down a series of passages that led me far into the back of the building. It was a maze with long halls going around corners and then bending back again. I was fairly certain that I had passed the same cork board twice. An old woman was standing near a short flight of stairs leaning on a broom and watching me.

"You look like you're lost." she said. "Whatcha looking for?"

"Park Unit," I told her.

"There ain't no Park Unit," she replied.

"I'm sorry. It's been a long day, I'm looking for the Adult Supervised Unit on the second floor," I said.

The old lady smiled knowingly and pointed at the stairs. "Go to the top, turn left and you'll walk right into it."

I thanked her and climbed the stairs. I felt about ninety years old. When I got to the top of the stairs, I turned left and nearly crashed into a door that was right in front of me. The door had frosted glass in the top panel and a doorbell ringer off to one side, with a hand-written message above it, in red ink. *Ring for entry.* Behind the frosted glass I could make out shadowy forms. I rang the bell. Almost immediately several dark forms approached the door from the other side. Then the door opened inward, and I heard a male voice say "Get back," and then "Just a minute." I didn't know if he was talking to me or to the other forms on his side of the door; so I waited to see what would happen next.

The door opened wider and someone said, "Well, come on; don't just stand there." I pushed in and found myself in another long corridor; only this time it was filled with people. Some had on white uniforms. Two such uniformed men were herding several individuals down the hallway. A woman I took to be the charge nurse stepped in front of me.

"Give me your purse and your coat," she said. These she handed over to another young man who had come out of a room that I assumed was an office, although it looked very unusual, having many shelves filled with cigarettes, hair spray and perfume, stockings and toilet paper.

"What patient are you here to visit?" She asked. She was holding a clip board, anticipating my answer. Her pen was poised, but I was having a hard time staying focused. I had become distracted by the young man who had started to rummage through my things. He had taken a cigarette lighter out of my purse and was placing it in a plastic bag.

"What the hell is going on here?" I asked her instead. She looked at me from over the tops of her glasses and sighed. Then she explained that they searched everyone's belongings for hair spray, cigarettes, matches, knives, fingernail files, and the like.

Apparently all of these things were potential hazards for people who had recently been trying to kill themselves. "This ward is restricted," she said. Suddenly I understood the contents of the shelves in the office.

"The patient's name?" She asked.

"Ben, his name is Ben," I said.

She looked down at her clip board again and then back to me. "I'll be sure to inform him that you came to visit, but you can't see him yet. He's still in isolation," she said.

"But I'm his mother," I told her.

"I'm sorry, but he can't have any visitors yet. Please call first next time."

Suddenly we were interrupted by a great ruckus down the hall. A young girl was trying to hit one of the men in the white uniforms. The nurse gave me her card, ignoring the commotion. "Here -is-the-number-for-the-hospital-and-the-extension-for-this-unit-and-it's-time-for-you-to-leave," she said all in one breath.

The young man came out from the strange little office carrying my purse and coat. These he handed over to me, and I was gently shoved back out the door with the frosted panel. It closed behind me with a great thud. I didn't know what else I could do; so I just went back down the stairs. I was met again by the old lady with the broom. "Merry Christmas," she said.

Chapter 10

May 2000

I awoke suddenly, hearing quite plainly an opera from above me. I listened briefly, long enough to realize the words were all in Italian: *l'aurora, di bianco vestita, gia luscious dischiude al gran sol...* I looked out the window and had to think for a minute where I was. Waking up can sometimes be confusing when you move all the time or when you are traveling; with me it had been the former.

I remembered that I was in my own bedroom, in the new apartment, in a little suburb, just outside of Baltimore. I had been living in the apartment for the last three months but hadn't got used to the surroundings yet. Sometimes I thought that I was still in the country and that when I got out of bed my old bathroom would be just down the hall. But now everything in my life had changed.

E. J. Cockey

There was an apple tree behind my apartment and a little rivulet just behind the tree. Beyond the tree and the stream there was a forest where birds were singing. I turned over in my bed and listened to the Italian songs from above, *Ove tu sei nasce l'amor...* *(Where you are love is born).* The clock radio came on, interfering with the opera from the neighbor's apartment. The announcer was saying that it's Sunday, 10 am, and the possibility for rain is slim to none. I sat up and turned the radio off. It was time to get up.

I tiptoed out into the living room, not sure whether Ben was sleeping or not. His bedroll was stuffed behind the couch; so I assumed that he was at work already. We were roommates now.

After he came home from the hospital, we stayed another six weeks with Evelyn; but the distance from the city was too great, and I had only my one car. Ben had gotten a job; so I drove him back and forth for a couple of months, but that got old after a while. Finally I was able to buy him a used car and wanted to begin paying off some of the medical bills. I needed another source of money, and the solution had been to teach a regular painting class to normal adults as my fund-raising effort. It had been Lewis's idea. I had been lamenting my lack of money, and he had said, "Why don't you teach an independent painting class?"

"Are you crazy?" I had asked him.

"Well, it's something you already know how to do," he explained.

"The last thing I need is one more student, normal or not!" I said. "What the hell do you think I do all week long?"

"What are your other options?" Lewis had asked me.
Of course he was right. I had had no other options at the time.

To complicate things, Richard had called and wanted to sign up for art lessons. At first, I had objected. I was worried that he was a married man, and very lonely. I knew this because he had driven out to visit me again while I was still living at Evelyn's house, right after the Christmas holidays. It was that particular afternoon when he had talked about his life and his unhappy marriage. It definitely explained a lot about him, like why he was spending weekends hiking in the country with dumb old Lewis, and paying random visits to me and Evelyn when he could have been eating brunch at the Hopkins Club back in town.

It sounded as if his wife was lonely too. She, however, was spending much of her time and Richard's money on facials, clothes, manicures, and visiting her psychiatrist twice a week. Richard told me that she was about as warm and fuzzy as a cold stone. He went into some detail about how she had achieved a type of outward perfection with the help of several plastic surgeries, but now had all the allure of an ill-tempered mannequin.

They lived in the best part of town, though, right down the street from the Professor and Gertrude, where all the little ducks and duck mommies hung out around the perfect ponds. What a life! Anyway, he had found out about the painting class from Lewis, and he wanted to sign up. "I'll pay you in advance," he had said. It was a tempting offer, too. He wanted to pay me in advance for the whole season!

"No Richard!," was my response.

Sometime the next day, Linda Sue called. "I think you should let Richard in the class," she informed me.

"He's unhappily married," I told her, "It could be a disaster."

"I talked with him; he needs a friend," she said.

E. J. Cockey

"I don't need any more friends with problems," I told her.

"All he does is go to work, and then he mulches," she said.

"What are you talking about?" I asked.

"He told me his main satisfaction in his spare time is working in the garden. He ordered ten cubic yards of mulch, and he spends all his time mulching the flower beds in that huge yard. He's lonely!" she said.

"No," I said.

"If he pays in advance you'll have enough money to pay off Ben's car," she said.

"You are so Jewish," I said.

"Be practical," she retorted. And so in the end, I relented and let Richard into the painting class. And now it was Sunday, and the class would be waiting for me at the local coffee shop where we gathered before driving out to the country together. I had four students: Jen, a normal college student type; her mother, Carolyn, a recovering alcoholic; Linda Sue, my best friend; and Richard, the unhappily married doctor, my new friend.

The class began every Sunday at 1pm. I met my students at Starbucks, and we would decide where to paint after we had all gotten our coffee. I liked the idea of the group making the decision. It was the best way for me to feel as if I were just along for the ride, and for them to begin to participate and become acquainted with one another.

I was moving slowly this particular morning, mostly because it seemed hot already, even though it was only May. I opened the window of my bed room to see how hot it was. I could hear the hum of a million bugs outside. I slammed the window shut quickly and went into my little kitchen to start the coffee.

By the time I had showered, dressed, and had a piece of toast, it was nearly 12:45pm. I hurried out the door, knowing that I would be about five minutes late and probably the last one there. I was right about both; my class was waiting outside in the parking lot.

They had gathered in a tight huddle, and everybody waved as I maneuvered my car into the lot. Very hot air came up in a wave from the pavement and met me head on when I climbed out of my car. It was oppressive. I was beginning to believe this class had been a bad idea in the first place: I would never listen to anyone else's advice again, most certainly not Lewis's. Now I was stuck performing as an art instructor for the next two hours, and worse, for the next two months!

Richard jaunted across the parking lot as I was unloading my car with an easel and paints. He was dressed in khakis as if he were going on some kind of safari, with a straw hat cocked to one side on his head. He also had a backpack and a folding chair which he was carrying in one hand and his French easel in the other.

Richard seemed happy to see me. I, on the other hand, was not happy to see anyone that day. I felt I was always in charge, that the burden of responsibility rested with me. Mostly I felt like a rundown entertainer, now acting in commercials instead of movies. I was tired of being an artist, and I wanted to go back to bed.

"Great to see you!" he called.

"Same," I responded.

Richard stopped just short of running into me. He dropped all of his gear on the pavement and leaned closer as if to hug me. I saw the inevitable and turned to one side just in time to avoid close personal contact. Instead, he ended up giving me a wet kiss on the side of my cheek.

"Knock it off, Richard," I said. "I'm your art teacher, not your girlfriend, remember?" I rubbed his kiss off with the side of my arm.

"I'm just happy to see you," he said.

I could see Jen, her mother and Linda Sue giggling behind him. "Just tone it down a little; we've got a fan club," I said, with a nod of my head towards the group. He turned around quickly and then back towards me again, probably realizing that everyone was amused.

"Gosh, sorry," he said.

"It's okay. These things happen," I told him. "Where are we going this afternoon?"

Before Richard could say another word, Linda Sue answered for him. She strode over and slapped me on the back. "How do you feel about north Baltimore county?" she asked. "I have a friend who lives down the road from St. James Church in Monkton, and he's got an awesome pond with ducks."

I looked at Richard. "Can we all fit in your car?" I asked.

"Let's go!" he said waving towards Jen and her Mom. And with that we were packing off to the country, all of us, together.

Chapter 11

June 2000

The weeks wore on, and my outlook improved, in spite of the initial attitude I had had about teaching another painting class only because I needed the money. I actually grew to enjoy the interaction with adults who were not impaired except that all of them were bored with their lives in a general, sub-clinical kind of way.

The five of us talked, and we painted some too. I found out that Jen's Mom had just recovered from a bout with cancer earlier that year. We all wanted to know how she had gotten through her ordeal.

"One day at a time," she said. "I learned that in my AA meeting."

Linda Sue hated her entire family. "They just don't get me," she said. "I'm different from them; they're all terrible workaholics."

"Excuse me, don't you receive a nice little stipend every year from a trust fund your mother set up?" I asked. "You don't have any worries."

"It doesn't matter if no one loves you," she replied.

We got to know each other in ways that we normally couldn't have in any other context. I honestly don't know if it was because we finally got into the right side of our brains by painting together, or we were just comforted by each other's sadness.

Richard was waiting for his wife to get a job. It wasn't clear to any of us what the significance of this was. It was Jen's Mom who finally put our queries about his wife to a halt. "More will be revealed," she said. More second-hand wisdom from AA. We decided to back off.

One day we had set up our easels in an alley behind some historic buildings, to paint images of their slow decay. The houses had fascinated me because of their ability to remain standing for the last 200 years despite the obvious lack of care. Whoever was supposed to have loved and cherished them had either forgotten, or been busy doing other things.

"It seems like such a waste of a life, not caring about other people or places, like this house," I commented.

It was just the two of us that particular day. Everybody else was on vacation; and it was the first time we had ever been alone together. I felt awkward and stupid, because it seemed more like a date than an art lesson; but Richard seemed as if he were light years away. It was hot, and the air was still and muggy. I was sweating. When he didn't comment about a waste of a life, I decided to change the subject.

"I'm going to raise the classes' tuition," I said. I waited to see if he had heard me or not. When he still didn't respond, I began to worry. I started to worry that it was a huge mistake coming out here at all, just him and me.

"My wife is still working on her resume'," Richard finally said.

"What do you mean?" I asked.

"She doesn't have any real experience," he said.

"Then why is she editing her resume'?" I asked. "I mean, it's not as if she has to go back to work. She enjoys a privileged life, doesn't she?"

"She feels unfulfilled now that the boys are going off to college," he said.

"What about you?" I asked.

"Oh, I have a good job," he said.

Richard pulled his shoulders back after making this statement, and stretched. He looked over at me then and shrugged. "Listen, my wife doesn't really care about me, only my paycheck. I'm the one who is unfulfilled. I want to leave, have a chance for romance, and live happily ever afterwards." he said.

"And you are waiting for her to find a job so you can do this?" I asked.

"It seems like the right thing to do," he replied.

I started to laugh. He was making very broad statements, and he was basing his decision on what his wife might or might not do. "What if she doesn't find a job?" I asked. "What if she doesn't want you to leave."

Richard frowned and put his paintbrush down. He looked like a deer staring into the headlights of a truck. He licked his lips several times before he spoke again. "When she finds a job," he corrected me, "I will leave the marriage. I want my life back."

"It's never a good time to leave," I said. "It will seem like a good time, and then it's Mother's Day, or someone's birthday, Christmas, a birth; Aunt Marge breaks her leg; you lose money in the stock market, or whatever. The truth is, it's never a good time to leave if you are waiting for something to happen."

"What would you do if you were in my circumstances?" he asked. I hate it when someone asks me a question about what I would or would not do, especially when my answer might influence an outcome that is none of my business. I hesitated, not knowing what to say. *I've put my foot into it this time,* I thought to myself.

"I'd stay married," I said. "I'd advise you to stay married if at all possible. Divorce is the worst thing you can do to yourself and your family, even if your kids are all grown up. Don't leave hoping that the grass is greener somewhere else, or with someone else. It seldom is."

Richard looked forlorn. He stepped back slightly from the canvas he had been working on and wiped his brush on the side of his jeans. When he looked back at me again I could tell that the wind had gone out of his sails. "You're right," he said. "When you don't care about anyone or anything, it's a terrible waste of a life."

"Richard, go home," I said. "Painting class is over for today."

The truth was that I intended never to see him again. I thought a lot about what it felt like to spend part of an afternoon with him, how comfortable it was just being there. He laughed at my jokes. He was calm and kind. He was married to someone else. I decided after we got into our separate cars that I was going to call him the following week and let him know that I had decided to end the class early. I was going to return the remainder of his tuition and end this strange friendship once and for all. I really was, but that's not what happened.

Several days later, two policemen knocked at my apartment door, looking for Ben. They had official papers from Collier county in Naples, Florida. The papers turned out to be a court injunction preventing Ben from visiting his son unless it could be substantiated that he had recovered and was under the care of a doctor. There were several pages of rules to be agreed to and then signed.

After they had gone, I read over all the papers. What I was going to need was an official doctor's statement about Ben's mental condition. I decided it would be simpler if I called Richard and asked if he would type a letter for me, rather than hunt down all the shrinks who had first seen Ben. After all, Richard probably knew more about Ben's medical condition than any of them, and he could also use that fancy doctor language to substantiate the facts. So, I called him, and he agreed.

"Why don't you come over now?" he asked.

"Are you sure this is a good time? I don't want to interrupt anything," I told him. What I really meant was that I didn't want to run into his wife. He must have sensed my concern because his answer was reassuring.

"My wife is out getting her hair done, and the maids are here cleaning," he said. "It's just me and the dog."

I knew he lived right around the corner from Gertrude, but I had never been on his street; and I was unprepared when I drove around the circular drive leading up to his house. The address was correct, but the house was a huge mansion, built mostly of gray and tan stone blocks. It rose like a church and was surrounded by lush gardens.

At first I thought I must have gotten the directions wrong, and I was getting ready to leave, when the front door opened and Richard came out. I climbed out of my car, all the while looking up at the mansion. "This is where you live?" I asked. I was incredulous. I knew he was well off, but I was completely unprepared for the opulence of the house and the grounds.

Richard ignored my surprise and grabbed the ornate bronze handle on the large wooden door. He pulled the door handle with a flourish and stood holding the door open for me.

"This way, madam."

I didn't say anything to him, just pushed by and found myself standing in a vestibule. In front of me was yet another door, paned with glass. Through it I could see into the front hallway.

Richard squeezed around me and opened the second door. "Come on in," he said.

Inside the air was cold in comparison to the summer heat outside. I was standing in the middle of a foyer. The floor was made from polished black and white squares of inlaid marble. In front of me was a harpsichord made of honey-colored wood, with a vase of fresh cut flowers placed on top. To one side a spiral staircase rose gracefully. There were portraits in gilded frames, probably ancestors, rising upwards along the wall with the stairs. I could hear a vacuum cleaner running somewhere in the distance. The house had a peculiar smell, like old church hymnals and furniture polish.

I looked off to my right and saw a sitting room with a fireplace at one end. Inside this room there were pieces of Victorian furniture, a red striped couch, formal armchairs, and more large oil paintings hanging on the walls. To my left there was a formal dining room and another fireplace. A huge crystal chandelier hung from the ceiling over the table with more fresh flowers in the middle of the table.

I had become immobilized. I couldn't find my voice, but I was able to think about Richard in a whole new way. I was actually standing in the middle of what seemed to be a rather perfect and extravagant life. Up until now, I had only seen him out in the countryside, painting, wearing khakis and old T-shirts with paint on them, just like me.

But, I wasn't like him. That much was obvious to me, standing in the foyer that day and smelling church hymnals. He had a family that was still intact, living in a mansion, in the best part of town where wives got to stay home and take care of their children, and dinner was served in a dining room that could seat twenty people.

He had a picture-perfect life. It was my life, not his, that had been taken away. I had worked since I was fifteen years old because I had to. I had earned degrees, but only for the purpose of earning a decent living, not because I was even remotely interested in a career path, or didn't feel fulfilled. What I had really wanted to do was grow a vegetable garden. Had anyone ever asked me? No. There was never time to think about such nonsense in a life that was all about surviving.

That day, standing in the foyer, I realized that I was the one who had been merely surviving. Even old Gertrude had a family. Families were important; they made all the difference in the world. I had had no one who really cared about me for years. I started to cry, right there, with the fresh flowers and Richard's ancestors watching me from their vantage point on the stairwell. My shoulders began to shake, and I threw my hands up over my eyes. I was suddenly ashamed to be me. As you might well imagine, Richard didn't understand at all what any of this was about. I must have looked like a lunatic.

"What is the matter?" he asked, wringing his hands in front of him.

"I'm an orphan!" I wailed, and burst into fresh tears.

Suddenly his arms were going around me; he was pulling me close. I looked up and there he was, crying right along with me. "What are you crying for?" I blubbered at him.

"I can't stand to see you in pain," he said.

"What possible difference can that make to you?" I asked.

"I love you," he said.

Chapter 12

April 2004

I followed the directions that the Professor had given me to the convalescent center where Gertrude was staying. It was mid afternoon, and the parking lot was crammed full with cars. It had rained earlier that morning, but the sun had just started to come out again. I drove around for several minutes hoping that someone would pull out, but in the end I parked illegally in the staff lot behind one of the main buildings. I knew from experience that no one would notice, or care for that matter.

The facility was being expanded and renovated. There were tall mounds of dirt and jumbles of wire fencing around the borders of the buildings. I could hear the drone of large engines somewhere in the background. Everything was busy, busy, busy. People were coming and going into the building from the street level, and I followed a small group into the lobby. Inside there was a large sign that gave instructions about where everything was located. It was all very confusing. I looked at this information for a few moments, and then went to the reception desk. A very bored-looking woman glanced up from a book she had been reading and absently asked me. "Wha ya need?"

"I need to locate the long term care unit," I said. "I'm here to see a patient." She pointed over her shoulder without even looking at me and said "Over there. "

I walked to the left side of the lobby where she had indicated, managed to get on the next elevator going up and got off on the second floor. I ended up asking for more directions from two other people before I finally found the unit where Gertrude was staying. I succeeded in maneuvering down several hallways and around one nurses' station before I found her room. The entire ward was dark and gloomy despite the restoration going on. I wondered to myself if they were going to turn on the lights. Was it always this dark in here? It reminded me of the first time I had met Gertrude, when I had walked down the hallway to her room at the Professor's house, how dismal her hallway had been too. It seemed as if it had all happened very long ago, and the thought saddened me now.

The door to her room was ajar, and I could see Gertrude sitting up in a chair. She was dressed, and her hair had been combed flat against her head. She looked different than I remembered her. For one thing, she was wearing clothes, and the nightcap was missing. In all the years we had been together, I had seen her only in a nightdress. She was staring straight ahead and didn't turn when I entered her room. The overhead light was off, but there was a large window on one side of the room, and the shade had been raised. Outside I could see a tree's branches and hear them scraping against the pane of glass. There were large pink buds at the end of each little branch. Inside the little room was devoid of ornament. There was a small cot, a nightstand, and of course the chair that Gertrude was sitting in.

I stepped gingerly in front of Gertrude, but she acted as if she didn't even know that I was there. She continued to stare straight ahead. Her eyes were glazed over, and she was holding a small towel that she kept putting up to her mouth. My eyes had adjusted to the light now, and I saw why she was using the towel. Gertrude was drooling.

"Hi Gertrude, it's me!" I startled her at first, but she began to squint and look me up and down, keeping the towel near her mouth the whole time. She didn't say anything; so I tried again.

"Do you remember me?" I asked. She shook her head yes.

"Paint," she said.

"Yes, we paint together. I'm your art teacher," I reminded her. She smiled, and I saw that her dentures had been removed. She was smiling up with pink gums and catching little rivulets of drool with the towel. Seeing her like this actually sickened me for a moment. She must have sensed my revulsion because suddenly tears came into her eyes, and she made an effort to speak again. She took the towel away from her face.

"I'm sorry," she said.

"Oh please, don't," I said. Then I dropped down on my knees in front of her, putting both of my hands into her lap. We were both crying now.

Finally I gathered myself and straightened up a bit. She was still holding my hands in hers, searching my face. My knees were going numb, but I stayed where I was. The linoleum floor was shiny and very hard. I looked around the room again. I noticed that the walls had been painted a neutral tan, and they were bare.

I wiped my eyes with the side of one hand that I had extracted from Gertrude's grasp. "We'll have to hang some of your paintings up," I said. She nodded in agreement as she looked around her room.

"Where am I?" she asked.

"You're at a long term care facility," I explained, "and you're going to stay here until you can go home again." I knew that this was a lie, but I couldn't bear to tell her that she would probably die here. Gertrude shook her head side to side.

"No," she said.

"Yes you will, Gertrude; you'll go home again soon."

"Troy Hill?" she asked.

I knew that she was referring to her lifelong home near Pittsburgh, in a row house, three doors down the street from Saint Anthony's Cathedral. The church was famous for its "stations of the cross" with life-sized statues depicting the passion of Jesus.

Bus loads of people came from all over the United States to see the stations of the cross there. Many of the visitors had touched the statue of Jesus over the years, wearing some of the paint off his features. Eventually, the church installed an alarm system to prevent this from happening, but every so often Gertrude would hear the alarm going off, and then she would exclaim, "Somebody's touching Jesus again!" She loved to tell me that particular story, over and over again, laughing all the while.

During our time together, she had told me many stories about her life and her family. Her real father had died of influenza in 1918, leaving her mother to take care of four small children. They had moved in with Gertrude's grandfather, and her mother had taken a job as a cook with a wealthy family in town. Within two years, her mother remarried a man who had lost his wife in the same epidemic. He had been left with two young children, who with the four from Gertrude's family, and two more of their own, made a grand total of eight mouths to feed. I used to question how they had managed, but Gertrude always described her life as happy, with stories about her brothers and sisters and their escapades. She never once spoke of herself as impoverished; instead she had been rich with family, church, and God in her life.

When we painted, she would always say to me, "Make it Good!" That phrase was one that her Grandfather had instilled in her from the time she was a little girl. She said that it was her motto in life and that she felt obliged to pass it on to me.

"If you do your best, you'll come out all right, no matter what," she would tell me. And then she would point her index finger straight up, saying, "and don't forget to pray."

I wondered how she would describe her life now. I also wondered if anyone would tell her the truth about her future. It was quite obvious that she was never going home again, not to her son's home, and definitely not to Troy Hill. I looked around her room again, at the empty walls and the hard linoleum floor. The tree outside was scratching at the window, bringing me back to the present. I had lied to her.

For the last eight years, my job has been to convince individuals who are suddenly hospitalized, dying, or demented, that they have something to live for; and I have done just that. I have transformed invalids and people with Alzheimer's disease into artists; the lame paint, the blind sing, and they do so right up until the day they die. Now I didn't know what I was going to say or do. Suddenly the answer was obvious.

I said a silent little prayer. *Help me, God, to know what to say to her.* As if in answer, and to my surprise, Gertrude asked another question.

"How is your life?"

The funny thing was that in all the years we had known each other, she had never once asked me about my life. She had always seemed more interested in telling her own stories, and I had let her. The truth was, she simply didn't know anything about me at all.

"My son Ben graduates from college this spring," I said. At this she nodded approvingly.

"Did you get married?" she asked.

"Yes, about two years ago."

Gertrude smiled. She waved her hand towards the door. "Then you can go home now," she said.

She closed her eyes and lay back in her chair. I waited a moment or two, but she looked as if she had gone to sleep. I stood up gradually and turned to look down at her for the last time. She looked peaceful, just as a saint should.

The End